Women's Wisdom

Natural Wellness Strategies for the Menopause Years

WOMEN'S WISDOM

NATURAL WELLNESS STRATEGIES FOR THE MENOPAUSE YEARS

LAUREL ALEXANDER

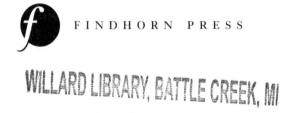

FINDHORN PRESS

Published in 2012 by Findhorn Press, Scotland

ISBN 978-1-84409-566-7

Edited by Nicky Leach
Cover design and illustrations by Richard Crookes
Interior design by Damian Keenan
Printed and bound in the EU

1 2 3 4 5 6 7 8 9 17 16 15 14 13 12

Published by
Findhorn Press
117-121 High Street,
Forres IV36 1AB,
Scotland, UK

t +44 (0)1309 690582
f +44 (0)131 777 2711
e info@findhornpress.com
www.findhornpress.com

CONTENTS

Disclaimer

The information in this book is given in good faith and is neither intended to diagnose any physical or mental condition nor to serve as a substitute for informed medical advice or care.

Please contact your health professional for medical advice and treatment. Neither author nor publisher can be held liable by any person for any loss or damage whatsoever which may arise from the use of this book or any of the information therein.

Introduction

What credentials do I have to write this book for you? I'm a complementary therapist and wellness coach with more than 15 years' experience in those fields, and a published author of numerous books on self-development and well-being. Particularly meaningful to me has been my work as a freelance complementary therapist for the UK's National Health Service (NHS), working alongside women going through the breast cancer journey (with particular emphasis on menopause). In addition—and maybe more importantly—I'm a 53-year-old woman and have irregular and heavy periods, mood swings (vulnerability, irritability, anxiety), vaginal itching, watery discharge, decreased libido, occasional insomnia, hot "flushettes," and occasional itchy skin. I've been travelling the perimenopausal journey for around three years now. Sometimes it's a pain in the butt, and sometimes I feel incredibly special.

Not only is my body changing but my inner landscape is shifting into new perspectives. I'm not so accepting of what others expect of me. I'm digging deeper into myself than ever before. Things that might have worried me once, I can't be bothered with now. I allow myself space. I speak my mind more often. I say no more frequently.

My interest in the philosophy of the Wise Woman Tradition spans many years. For me, the weave of ancient eclectic beliefs and values combined with practical application and modern psychology has provided a natural pathway through the apparent chaos of menopause. What a fantastic journey of change and opportunity it is proving to be! I'm up and down—both courageous and vulnerable, vaguely blank or teeming with creative ideas for change, withdrawn into retreat or at the hub of social gatherings. I'm both hidden and transparent in my Wise Woman pathway.

In this book, I would like to share with you some of the self-help tools you may like to work with on your special journey through the menopause years. Choose instinctively, and travel with Spirit.

—Laurel

A Wysecraft Tale for
the Menopause Years

The Dark Goddess stirs her coils in the blackness of the deepest dark and sends forth her handmaiden, the Wise Woman, to walk with all women on their journey of Change. This is what the Wise Woman whispers in your heart:

There you are—being in the community, caring for others, indulging in hobbies and crafts, laughing and crying with friends, engaging in domesticity, earning money to keep hearth and home together, moving with the ups and downs of life, ebbing and flowing on the tide of Doing.

You notice a change in your behavior or mindset. Something happens to make you look again. Your spiritual center of gravity is shifting out of the familiar to shadowy realms. What has always worked no longer seems to work as well. The nourishment from personal interactions seems unfulfilling. Activities that once fired you with passion are beginning to leave you arid and dry. Your life no longer nourishes you. You are missing a sense of connection. It may be an emotional quagmire, a practical challenge, a cognitive mish-mash, or a spiritual crisis. Destiny is calling you. You are moonstruck woman. This is the time of dark blood—the time of menopause.

You feel pinpricks of fear. What is this? What is happening? What is life about for you if this or that, him or her, no longer seem to give meaning to your life? There is fragmentation, as parts of your life seem to fall away. There is a desire to run into the past and hide behind memories of the familiar. You pretend all is well as your inner landscape shifts beneath the feet of your daily life. You pretend to hold things together to avoid falling into some kind of spiritual abyss. You lean on psychological and physical compulsions. You ignore the call, throwing yourself into a frenzy of activities that hold little meaning in their illusion of safety as you slip towards the unknown.

All is the same. ALL IS WELL. If you shout loud enough, you believe you can drown out the voices—the fear and the loneliness as you move into what seems to be permanent night. Your distress is the beginning of your journey back to Self through the landscape of menopause.

I am your Wise Woman, your internal teacher. I will guide you through this transformative journey, as you begin to seek the knowledge that is within you. I will be present in your deepest despair. I will nurture you in the dark, as you descend into the shadow of your psyche. I will connect you to the awakening of your power and your creative fire.

As you walk through this symbolic inner world, you will interact with others in your daily life—both people you know and people you don't know—who can help you face the unknown. Day by day, you move towards your first rite of passage. You meet the symbolic guardians of your inner dimensions. They will try to prevent your entry to the realms of self-discovery. At work or in your private life, these guardians will appear as well-meaning people who press your buttons of self-doubt.

You will face them with courage and pass through the inner gate, a mindset activity, which may be reflected in the outside world through changing life circumstances. You have committed yourself to finding out your authentic nature and what your life needs to be. Crossing the threshold is your first step into the sacred realm of the Dark Goddess, which will take you to the source of all mysteries. I, your Wise Woman, will teach you how to experience yourself profoundly, how to be creative, assertive, intuitive, and sexual. You will face tests in your life, meeting foes and trusted companions along the road.

In a symbolic sense, you are journeying deep into the forest to regain your power and wholeness. The country you travel through is hazardous, dark, and filled with the unknown. You may experience work challenges, health issues, family difficulties, limited finances, and a loss of purpose or relationship problems.

How you relate to yourself and express your potential will change. New people will cross your path, and you will be exposed to fresh ideas. You will renew your relationship with nature and the subtle dimensions of mind and spirit. With each new difficulty you embrace, you will develop inner strength, greater knowledge, and increased power for what lies ahead. You will collect more support from companions who will be useful in your purpose as you approach the most dangerous place of all—the innermost cavern of your being. Deeper into the forest and down into the underworld you travel.

Here is the nucleus of your journey—the inner sanctum of the Dark Goddess. You are approaching a time for solitude in this inner realm. You find your nemesis in the uterine-like cave where the Dark Goddess resides. The Dark Goddess is the symbolic initiator of menopause. She lives at your core. She is the midwife of your soul. She will guide you into a new way of living through a symbolic rebirth. She will move you through the cauldron of destruction of all that you no longer need to a place of authentic clarity.

You may become aware of soul loss during the menopause years—a feeling of disassociation and joylessness. Within this womb-like cave, you need to listen and learn before you can find the misplaced part of your soul, your treasure of knowledge and self-discovery. You will feel confused, grief-stricken, despairing, lonely, and angry. The darkness within the symbolic winter earth chills you to your core. Outside the cave, deep underground, you can hear the distant roar of volcanic activity as life continues to teem and foment with passion. As you walk through your spiral of transformation, now is the time to probe the mysteries of decay and regeneration. You will feel raw and vulnerable as you plunge to your core of truth. What roles are you hiding behind in your life? Have your ambitions been yours or someone else's? Are you selling your soul for the apparent kudos it might buy? To what extent have you bargained away your passion for what you think will bring you safety? Whose fears are you trying to placate by ignoring your own dreams? How do your self-deceptions manifest? There will be no comfort in the underworld as you hear and answer these questions.

As the moon grows to the deepest black and your bleeding slows, the Dark Goddess settles within your being. Instead of the menstrual flow, your dark blood of power is retained for creative use. The Dark Goddess is the destroyer of all that seeks to separate you from your essential nature. She demands that you clear out of your life all that is no longer essential, all that does not help you grow or help you fulfill your deepest needs.

You have turned within to know your mind with its enmeshment of thought and feeling, your body with its desires, and your spiritual needs. You have moved into your shadow depths to reclaim parts of yourself that have been lost. You have faced the supreme ordeal and confronted your greatest fears. You have undergone a symbolic life and death moment—the core challenge of your journey. The Dark Goddess is the High Priestess of Death and Regeneration. In the role of midwife, she has assisted in your rebirth to a new way of being. It is over, and the Dark Goddess blesses you and gives you the greatest treasure of all: your soul. Symbolically, you wear nothing but the all-encompassing deepest purple cloak, which represents the gateway between matter and spirit, as you begin to take your true place in the reality of your daily living.

Nature is your balm. Your spirit is fed by the earth. A stream that begins from deep within the earth's core releases its coolness into the cave and beyond. It will lead you out of the underworld to the land above with soul intact and in a transformed state. Now you need to bring yourself back to your daily life. Be aware. Old shadows murmur their seductive ways. Worn ideas and meaningless ways of doing things whisper their call to you.

But you have changed. A spiritual alchemy has taken place within you. You need to learn new ways of being and doing as you return from the underworld to your new life above. The old ways no longer work. You will experience a testing of your new powers as your soul takes rebirth and emerges from the womb, a new creature.

You will need your body to be cleansed inside and out and recharged with positive energy. You will need a refocus of your outer life to reflect the inner changes. There is new joy, new meaning. There is knowledge of integration, personal power, and freedom. You are the mistress of your own life. You engage in "creative doing," because the desire to do so springs from your true nature.

These are the Wysecraft words for working with your menopause years:

- Honor your instincts, and set your intentions;
- Allow your relationships with others to deepen;
- Create ritual in your life;
- Stretch your vision, and express your core energy in life;

- Trust yourself;
- Make daily time to be alone and to restore yourself;
- Become aware of your energy shifts (physical, psychological, and subtle);
- Don't allow others to drain or live off your energy;
- Free yourself from harmful beliefs;
- Don't live off others' energy;
- Transmute negative energy (yours and others);
- Engage in creative self-expression.

I am your Wise Woman through the menopause years and beyond, until your physical body passes from this dimension of consciousness to the next. I will always walk by your side. May the blessing of the Dark Goddess be with you throughout all time.

CHAPTER 1

Moving Through Menopause

Today, menopause is seen as a gateway to a second adulthood and marks a midway point in our life. A century ago, the average age of menopause was 47, but life expectancy was only 49. According to Dr Annie Evans, woman's health specialist at the Bristol Royal Infirmary in Britain, with life expectancy now set at almost 80, women today are becoming menopausal around 50 years of age, living an additional 30 years following menopause. [1]

The term "baby boomer" is applied to people born between 1946 and 1964. During this time the economies of most nations boomed, leading people to feel greater confidence in having babies. This generation, has challenged many sociological traditions, including menopause. According to *Baby-Boomer* magazine (2010), [2] a baby boomer turns 50 every seven seconds. Many women entering and going through their menopause years are realizing they can experience their journey with a positive attitude and good health.

The word "menopause" comes from the Greek word *pausis* (cessation) and means "end of monthly cycles" and the root *men-* (month). The menopausal transition is a natural life change and part of aging, signaling the end of your reproductive years in a child-bearing sense. Natural menopause occurs in the following stages:

STAGE ONE: Perimenopause (late 30s – late 40s)

This term is used to describe the first stage of the process in which there are significant changes to your hormone levels leading to menopause. Estrogen and progesterone—hormones made by your ovaries that are responsible for fertility—naturally begin falling during perimenopause.

This impacts your reproductive ability and menstrual cycle, causing the typical signs of fluctuating hormones, such as irregular, scant, or heavy periods due to skipped ovulations. The duration of flow may be shorter or longer than normal, and the flow itself may be heavier or there may be occasional spotting. Periods eventually become lighter and less frequent due to decreased egg production by the ovaries. Early in the process, it is not uncommon to have some two-week cycles. Farther into the process, it is common to skip periods for months at a time, and these skipped periods may be followed by a heavier period. The number of skipped periods in a row often increases as the time of last period approaches. Note: Irregular or heavy bleeding can be caused by conditions other than menopause, such as fibroids or polyps.

Early perimenopause

Symptoms of perimenopause can begin as early as 10 years before menstruation stops. In addition to irregular menstrual cycles, you are likely to experience:

- Cramps
- Weight gain
- Headaches
- Emotional shifts
- Thinning of the membranes of the vulva, vagina, cervix, and outer urinary tract, due to low estrogen levels, as well as, potentially, vaginal itching and dryness, watery discharge, and decreased libido.

The bodies of both men and women produce the follicle-stimulating hormone (FSH), which is the hormone produced by the pituitary gland. It stimulates the production of sperm in men and production of eggs in women, and releases the hormone estradiol in the early stages of the menstrual cycle. FSH normally surges about 24 to 36 hours before the release of an egg as part of the menstrual cycle, which is then either fertilized or eliminated from the body during a period. Estrogen levels peak at about the same time, then decrease, with another smaller peak in the second half of the menstrual cycle, while progesterone levels start rising at this time. FSH levels fall after their mid-cycle peak and remain at a steady level until nearly the end of that cycle.

In women, high levels of FSH can be an indication that your ovaries are shutting down egg production, meaning that menopause has started. A drop in estrogen levels forces up levels of FSH, which serves as a reminder for the ovaries to produce eggs, but now the ovaries are unresponsive, leading to further increases in FSH levels. Note: High levels of FSH may also be the sign of underlying disease. You may still be fertile at this time, although it may be difficult to become pregnant due to an irregular ovulation cycle that will eventually end.

Late perimenopause

The late stages of perimenopause involve more noticeable changes in the body, as your ovaries reduce hormonal production even further. This stage in the process is characterized by a woman experiencing a range of physical and psychological symptoms right up until the date of her last period. These symptoms include:

- Insomnia, fatigue, and lethargy caused by low levels of estrogen (exacerbated by night sweats) or brought on by anxiety or depression;
- Tendency to feel anger;
- Depression—more likely in the years immediately before menopause, especially if you've experienced premenstrual syndrome (PMS) in the past;
- Anxiety/panic attacks;

- Hot flushes and night sweats, which occur as the felt body temperature soars. The sensation of heat is not in response to a temperature rise but a reaction to the slowness of the body's return to a normal temperature range. Symptoms associated with hot flushes (called vasomotor symptoms, as they involve nerves and muscles that cause blood vessels to constrict or dilate) include: feeling of intense heat in body or on the face, palpitations, dizziness, nausea, headache, weakness, anxiety, feeling trapped or suffocated, a tingling sensation of the skin (formication), and flushed appearance or blotchy skin;
- Dry or itchy skin, due to thinner skin (without estrogen, our skin finds it difficult to retain moisture);
- Bladder problems, such as cystitis or other bladder infections; reduced bladder capacity; and stress incontinence caused by loss of muscle and tissue elasticity in the pelvic cavity, leading to a tendency to leak urine on laughing or coughing;
- Vaginal changes (as noted above).

Conditions affecting perimenopause

If a woman's body has been impacted by poor nutrition, such as consuming inadequate protein and too many carbohydrates, inadequate essential nutrients and fats, excess drinking, chronic stress, smoking, long-term exposure to environmental toxins and artificial hormones, or a lack of regular exercise over the proceeding years, this seems to make the perimenopausal symptoms stronger.

When I was 39, I was diagnosed with estrogen-receptive breast cancer (meaning the more estrogen my body produced, the more aggressively the cancer could grow). I chose to go on the drug tamoxifen for five years. According to the National Cancer Institute at the National Institutes of Health in the United States, tamoxifen inhibits the production of estrogen [3] and can put premenopausal women into a sudden and abrupt early menopause. However, the blessings I had were that my periods became regular, shorter, lighter, and pain-free!

At 53, I'm in the late stages of perimenopause. My main issue is unpredictable periods with occasional flooding in the early bleed. My mother tells me how her mother, my grandmother, used to flood onto the kitchen floor! Umm, not the more reassuring of images! My sister, who is six year older than me, is postmenopausal and tells me of how dreadful her flooding was while she was going through the mid to late perimenopausal stage. Getting panicky now! However, there are many pathways in Wise Woman healing, and I create my own reality (as you do) with each loving step. I would like to add that flooding can also occur for other reasons, such as fibroids. If you are at all concerned, please get yourself checked with a qualified healthcare professional.

Early menopause

While the total number of women with early menopause represents a small percentage of the female population, statistics may not be accurate because many aspects of early menopause overlap with premature ovarian failure (POF). Women can also move more quickly into menopause after undergoing certain kinds of surgery or medical treatments. Here are some common terms used to classify menopause: [4]

- *Surgical menopause* occurs as a result of hysterectomy, oophorectomy (removal of ovary/ovaries), and some other pelvic surgeries.
- *Medical menopause* can occur following medical treatments such as radiotherapy and chemotherapy, and during the course of drug regimens like tamoxifen. In some cases, fertility may return after treatment ends.
- *Premature ovarian failure (POF)* is a medical expression

used to describe loss of ovarian function in women younger than 40.

Other reasons could include autoimmune diseases, such as lupus, diabetes, and rheumatoid arthritis, or infectious diseases like malaria. Medical conditions that can cause menopausal symptoms include thyroid disorders and other endocrine disorders.

The symptoms of early menopause are essentially the same as those for perimenopause and menopause. In addition, issues around the loss of fertility can make early menopause a particularly bittersweet time.

> **WISE WOMAN WAYS**
>
> Menopause is likely to occur for us at the same age as it did for our mothers. If your mother's menopause was early, yours may be, too.

STAGE TWO: Menopause (50s)

The menopausal transition leads to the permanent termination of a woman's period and her fertility, otherwise known as the Change. In women who have a uterus, menopause is medically defined as having taken place if a menopausal woman has not had a period for 12 months.

The menopausal passage is determined as having been completed with the natural or surgical cessation of the production of estradiol (the most potent of the three forms of estrogen in the body) and progesterone by the ovaries. After menopause, a weaker form of estrogen (estrone) continues to be produced in much smaller amounts in the ovaries and adipose tissue (body fat), while progesterone levels drop dramatically, with small amounts continuing to be produced in the adrenal glands and stored in adipose tissue.

The menopausal climax years include the year or two before and a year or more after your very last menstruation. The average age of the last menstruation is 51. During this time, the bones refuse to take in calcium, and bone scans may show the preliminary stage of osteoporosis, known as osteopenia; hot flushes and night sweats may be frequent; palpitations, emotional sensitivity, and sleeplessness are common.

STAGE THREE: Postmenopause

The term "postmenopause" refers to women who have not had a menstrual bleed for at least one year, (assuming that they are not pregnant). In women without a uterus, postmenopause is identified by a high FSH level. Postmenopause is all of the time in a woman's life that follows the point when her ovaries become inactive.

Being postmenopausal doesn't mean hormone withdrawal symptoms will disappear straight away. Reproductive hormone levels continue to drop and fluctuate, and symptoms may take time to disappear. Due to a decline in estrogen and as a result of aging, this stage brings with it a new set of health issues, such as heart disease and strokes and osteoporosis, leading to thinning bones and an increase in fractures, particularly in the hip or spine, and cancer.

There are many things to celebrate about being postmenopausal. No more bleeding or hot flushes. No more worry about pregnancy. Now you can find your real voice and make positive changes that will take you forward in your life.

WISE WOMAN WAYS
Any period-like flow that might occur during postmenopause (if you are not undergoing hormone replacement therapy), even just spotting, must be checked out by a qualified medical person.

Psychology of the Menopausal Years

Anxiety, depression, sadness, difficulty concentrating, overreacting to minor upsets, anger, irritability, panic attacks, forgetfulness, and mood swings are all typical of the psychological issues we may face during the menopause years. Some symptoms will be hormone-related, while others are due to the changes in a woman's life around that time.

Situations and life events that tend to crowd into a woman's life in her late 40s and 50s include [5] having to deal with caring for and/or the death of elderly parents, birth of grandchildren, children leaving home, divorce, retirement of self or partner, widowhood, and altered self-image due to aging. Other psychological challenges can include beliefs about no longer being useful, distorted body image, fear of death, feeling unemployable, low self-worth, and a sense of loss related to the end of fertility.

WISE WOMAN WAYS

Across indigenous cultures, such as the Iroquois and Navajo (North America), the Maori (New Zealand), some African cultures, and the women of traditional shamanic cultures, such as the Cree (Canada) and the Maya, there is a common belief that women entering menopause can access their healing and shamanic powers. The power of menstrual blood creates life in the womb, and when women reach the age of retaining their "wise blood," they become a "wise woman" and spiritual elders of their communities.

Jubilee

The Jubilee study (named for the female experience before and after the age of 50) was carried out by the Social Issues Research Centre in the United Kingdom and commissioned by HRT Aware. [6] The study surveyed some 200 postmenopausal women aged 50-64 in the UK and found that, following menopause:

- 65 percent of them were happier than prior to menopause;
- 66 percent felt greater independence;
- 59 percent said their relationships with friends and partners had improved;
- 48 percent reported that their working lives had improved at postmenopause;
- 29 percent claimed sex was better than ever.

The typical woman surveyed was middle class, well educated, and knowledgeable about health issues. The published report states that the participants represented, "a new elite, nicknamed HRH's—'hormone-rich and happy.'"

What Happens Next?

As we can see, there are medically defined stages as we move through menopause. But when we look at menopause through Wise Woman eyes, we move away from the scientific way of understanding this change in a woman's life into the profoundly empowering realms that can help us celebrate the rites of passage to the Dark Goddess. Read on to discover your connection with the Dark Goddess.

CHAPTER 2

Celebrating the Dark Goddess

In order to understand the relevance of the Wise Woman during the menopause years, we need to get a sense of how the Goddess belief system developed through history and across the cultures of the world.

Hunter-Gatherer Societies

Until about 8,000 BC, our ancestors organized themselves into hunter-gatherer societies [7] with religious beliefs that revolved around their land-based lifestyle. Hunting was pivotal to tribal survival, and as a result, the hunter element in society (mostly men) tended to worship hunting gods and animals, such as the God of the Hunt or the Stag Horned God (or buffalo).

Women were mostly the gatherer element in society. They took care of the tribe and were the child bearers and healers. The female life-giving principle was considered divine, and the importance of fertility and birthing in crops, animals, and in the tribe itself was crucial to survival. As a result, women in hunter-gatherer societies tended to worship vegetative goddesses. While men and women might have worshipped similar gods and goddesses within the tribal community, they may also have gravitated to gender specific worship. Women experienced a connection between their bodies and the phases of the moon that further enhanced the mystical link with the moon and the Goddess deity. Because of these links, women during this time tended to lead the spiritual rituals of the tribe.

As society evolved, people began to settle in one place, growing food and breeding animals. This was when they became paganized (the word "pagan" is derived from the Latin word *paganus,* meaning "country dweller"). Paganism originates from the Neolithic (Stone Age) era. It was thought that everything had a spirit, so people had gods and goddesses for all aspects of their lives including nature. Civilizations developed, and the gods were adapted to the changing lives of the people to play an important role in every aspect of the community.

The Goddess Influence

The word "goddess" means a female divine being. Around the world for thousands of years, many societies have worshipped a divine and powerful Mother-Goddess, and goddess images of great antiquity have been found all over the world. Several small, figures have been found during archaeological excavations of the Upper Paleolithic, such as the Venus of Willendorf [8] (24,000–22,000 BC). These figures are typical of a postmenopausal female body.

Cave paintings and rock carvings of goddesses have been found that date back to 35,000 years BC or earlier. Early humans noticed all life was created within the bodies of women, and so it was natural for them to see an all-powerful creator as female, too. Many cultures around the world still worship goddesses. For example, many Christian traditions offer blessings that include the Mother. Inuit people honour the Ocean Mother Sedna. Quan Yin (Goddess of Mercy) is honoured by many Chinese. And Hindus have many goddesses in their tradition.

The Triple Goddess

Long before the advent of Christianity, the Temple in Jerusalem had a tower representing the Great Goddess in her triple aspect. Known as Mari (a possible ancient goddess source influencing the later worship of Mary and the Virgin Mother), the images shown are the three stages of the female life cycle: the premenstrual maiden, the fertile menstrual nymph, and the postmenopausal crone. [9]

Neopagan [10] is a broad definition used for a wide variety of modern religious or spiritual concepts influenced by the pre-Christian pagan beliefs of Europe. Wicca (popularly called White Witchcraft, the benign religion of the ancient Celts and an example of neopaganism) reemerged in the mid-20th century in England. Not only does Wicca tend to honour the Triple Goddess of maiden (virginity), mother (fertility), and crone (wisdom)[11] but it also honours the Horned God. These two deities are often viewed as being a sacred blend of nature (or the universe) and the Divine. The Maid-Mother-Crone symbolizes the following:

- The Maid of childhood and adolescence: youth and possibility, emerging sexuality;
- The Mother of child-bearing years: creativity and nurturing;
- The Crone of the menopausal years: wisdom transition, the compassion that comes from experience, and the one who guides us through the death and rebirth experience.

Each phase of the Triple-Goddess—maiden, mother, and crone—represents a different type of healing and growth in a woman's life. Her aspects are mirrored in the phases of the moon: new, waxing, full, and waning. This goddess philosophy linking spirituality and earth cycles can be found across many timeframes and cultures, including Norse, Greeks, Hindu, Celtic, and Roman belief systems.

The Maiden, Mother, and Crone aspects represent linear life cycles while, simultaneously, each stage can be found within the other stages. For example, I can identify with the idea of a Triple Goddess. At 53, I'm a Crone; however, I can (when the mood takes me) become a Maiden, and although I am not a physical mother, my Mother instincts often come out with partner, family, friends, students, and clients.

The Dark Goddess of the Menopause Years

Menopause is symbolically the initiation of the Dark Goddess, and the archetypal spokeswoman for the Dark Goddess is the Crone (or Wise Woman). At this time, we confront our own mysteries of transformation as the Dark Goddess dissolves old patterns of thinking, feeling, and behaving; acting as midwife, she gives birth to new ways. During the menstrual years, at the dark of each monthly moon, she comes to release your life blood. As you move through menopause, the Dark Goddess stays within your core; the dark blood now retained within your body for transformation into creative energy. She is the teacher who guides you through the process of Change. Examples of Dark Goddess from around the world include: [12]

Africa

ALA: Earth Mother Goddess of the Ibo tribe in Nigeria. Creator of the Living and Queen of the Dead. Provider of communal loyalty and lawgiver of society.

ASASE YAA: Old Woman Earth of the Ashanti people of western Africa. She gave birth to humanity and reclaims her children at death. At planting, the Ashanti farmer prays to his ancestors and to Asase Yaa, who lent the rights of cultivation to the living.

Celtic: Britain, France, and Spain

ARIANRHOD: Mother Goddess of Celtic Aryans and Keeper of the endlessly circling Silver Wheel of the Stars (symbol of time).

BRANWEN: Goddess of Regeneration who kept the Cauldron of Regeneration.

CAILLECH: Old Celtic name for Kali, the Great Goddess in her destroyer aspect. The Veiled One. Great pre-Celtic goddess of the British Isles.

MORGAN LE FAY: Death Goddess.

China

MAT CHINOI: Serpent Goddess. Mother of the Chinese. In her belly lived beautiful angels who received the souls of the dead.

Ancient Crete

CIRCE: Death Goddess.

HECATE: Moon Goddess. Protector of childbirth. Wise Crone of the Hebe. Goddess of Magic and Prophecy. Goddess of the Dark Moon.

MAIA: White Goddess. Greek goddess of the spring and rebirth. As the mother of Hermes, she was considered the Grandmother of Magic.

PERSEPHONE: Queen of the Underworld. Destroyer Goddess. Crone of the Triple Goddess with Kore and Demeter.

CROWNED BUTTERFLY GODDESS (4,000 BCE): Arising from the horns of the sacred bull, this Minoan Crowned Butterfly Goddess symbolized fertility and regeneration.

India and Tibet

KALI: Black Earth Mother. Goddess of fertility, death, and regeneration. Dark Mother. Hindu Triple Goddess of creation, preservation, and destruction. Birth and Death Mother. A triple Goddess: Maiden, Mother, Crone. Lady of the Dead.

SMASHANA-KALI: Kali Ma. Goddess of cremation grounds and other places of Death. The word means "Rebirth following Death".

UMA: The Golden Goddess, personifying light and beauty. Kali's Crone aspect.

Japan

FUJI: Grandmother. Ancestor. Holy Mother Mountain.

Rome

COVENTINA: Mother of Covens. Celtic goddess as patroness of healing wells and springs.

PROSERPINA: Queen of the Underworld.

Maya and Aztec – Mexico

COATLICUE: Lady of the Serpent Skirt. Mother of all Aztec deities, as well as the Sun, Moon, and Stars. She produced life and received the dead.

MICTECACIUATL: Eponymous Mother Goddess of Mexico. Lady of the Place of the Dead.

TLAZOLTEOTL: Aztec Mother Goddess resembling the medieval Hecate as Queen of the Witches. She was associated with the Moon.

Middle East

SHAYBA: Arabic-Aramaean title of the Great Goddess. Shayba was Old Woman, whose spirit dwelt in the Sacred Stone of the Kaaba in Mecca.

North America – Southwest

SPIDER GRANDMOTHER: Goddess creator of the world in Native American religions and that of the Navajo and Pueblo cultures. She wove the universe every day and unraveled the web every night.

Norse/Teutonic – Northern Europe

FREYA: Great Goddess of northern Europe. Mediator between peace and violence, she presided over the living and the dead.

HALJA: Gothic name for Hel, Goddess of the Underworld.

HEL: Norse Queen of the Underworld. Goddess of the Dead.

SKADI: Celto-Teutonic goddess in her destroyer aspect. Queen of the Shades, Mother Death.

Polynesia

PELE: Hawaiian Goddess of Fire and the Underworld.

Russia/Slavic

BABA YAGA: Crone Goddess.
MARZANNA: The personification of Death and Winter.
MORENA: Slovakian Goddess of Death and Regeneration.

Other Goddesses

BENDIS: (Thrace) Goddess of Destruction, the Crone, and the Waning Moon.
MARA: (India) Exceedingly ancient name of the Goddess-as-Crone, the Death-bringer.
NINHURSAG: (Akkadia) Goddess who is Mistress of Serpents. She Who Gives Life to the Dead.

> **WISE WOMAN WAYS**
>
> How you might choose to relate to the concept of the Dark Goddess is a very personal thing. When I'm teaching students about the Goddess concept, I give the metaphorical idea of a multifaceted crystal and the different facets as the female presenting all her different sides (or faces, roles, and masks). Consider your own sense of femaleness. What roles and masks do you present? Which are authentic and which are fixed on by duty or responsibility or to please someone else? The Dark Goddess is our shadow side, the hidden facets of our female nature that we fear or believe we should have shame about, but in reality is our release mechanism to transmute darkness into light.

Maybe it's because I'm a Scorpio, or maybe it's just that it's in my soul to plumb the depths, but I love the imagery and experience of the Dark Goddess. Wrapping the metaphorical cloak of darkness around me and withdrawing into the depths (in bite-sized chunks) nourishes me when "out there" becomes overwhelming. Having said that the depths can be overwhelming as well, so there needs to be a balance—always a balance.

Cronehood and the Menopause Years

The Crone is the Wise Woman or grandmother. She is both midwife and healer. In human years, she is approximately 45 years of age or older. Her profound and evolving wisdom gives her grace and dignity. The colour purple is associated with the time of croning. When purple clothing or jewellery is worn by a menopausal woman, it indicates she is owning her Wise Womanhood.

The Wise Woman cares for both Maiden and Mother. She represents death and rebirth, the transforming of endings into beginnings. Life events involving the Wise Woman include menopause, aging, moving home, retribution, ending of relationships or activities, rest before making new plans, nature moving into winter, and the great mysteries of life, death and rebirth.

The Wise Woman is the mistress of wisdom, retrenchment, repose, and compassion and was revered in ancient cultures as a representative of the Underworld, a place where souls went to rest between incarnations, before coming back to the earthly plane.

What Happens Next?

We can see that the journey through menopause can be full of inner symbolism. Working with this can help us to make some sense of our spiritual and psychological journey. Just as we need to learn about and nourish our inner Wise Woman, we mustn't forget to nourish our physical body through good nutrition. The next chapter sets out recommended supplements and foods for a range of menopausal symptoms.

Useful Resources

- *www.birthingthecrone.com* (a wonderful site showing the work of artist Helen Redman).
- *www.cronemagazine.com* (for women of all spiritual paths, *Crone is* an advertising-free 128-page magazine published twice yearly in the UK in both paper and PDF eZine formats).

CHAPTER 3

Good Nutrition

Good food provides not only goodness for mind and body but also supplies the raw materials your neuroendocrine (nerve-hormone) system needs to create healthy hormonal and emotional balance as you go through menopause.

Progesterone and Menopause

Progesterone is the hormone produced by the female ovaries after ovulation. It supports and maintains pregnancy, is the precursor to other vital hormones, and is needed to balance estrogen levels. Estrogen promotes cell growth, and progesterone keeps that growth from going farther than is healthy. Your estrogen levels may be unbalanced if your body is not producing enough progesterone.

Most women begin to produce less progesterone in their early 30s, and this loss accelerates in their 40s. After menopause, the female body hardly makes any progesterone, although women continue to make estrogen throughout their lives. This progesterone deficiency causes several symptoms of perimenopause.

The use of bioidentical or natural progesterone cream to treat female hormonal issues was pioneered by the late Dr. John Lee, [13] a Californian family doctor. It is made in the laboratory from plant sources such as Mexican yam and, as the term "bioidentical" indicates, it is identical to the hormone produced by the ovaries. Natural progesterone can be used to help support menopausal issues, such as irregular menstrual flow, bloating, depression, irritability, insomnia, hot flushes, vaginal dryness, and low sex drive.

NOTE: Bioidentical progesterone cream is readily available over the counter in a basic strength in health food stores like Whole Foods in the United States, as well as by specific-strength prescription from your doctor through special compounding pharmacies. The situation in the United Kingdom is different, however. Bioidentical progesterone cream is not licensed for medical use in the United Kingdom, and as a result, is only available as an unlicensed medicine by prescription from your doctor. If you choose not to consult a doctor, you can legally import bioidentical progesterone cream from outside the United Kingdom, provided it is solely for your own use. Several well-known companies, such as Emerita, make their products available in the United Kingdom. [14]

> **WISE WOMAN WAYS**
>
> Agnus castus is said to work at the level of the pituitary gland and can increase progesterone production. Take it consistently for a few months in tincture form. Evening primrose may boost progesterone levels although its main role is balancing both progesterone and estrogen and bringing them to their correct levels.

Phytoestrogen Foods

Phytoestrogens are weak estrogen-like compounds in plants (*phyto* means plant). They lock onto and block estrogen receptors, making it harder for harmful chemicals to disrupt hormone signals. It is thought that phytonutrients act as hormone regulators, rather than mimicking estrogen or progesterone.

Food sources include oats, barley, rye, brown rice, couscous, bulgar wheat, sunflower seeds, sesame seeds, pumpkin seeds, poppy, linseeds, tofu, soy products (except soy sauce), citrus, chickpeas, kidney beans, haricot beans, broad beans, green split peas, red onions, green beans, celery, sweet peppers, garlic, broccoli, tomatoes, rhubarb, apples, aniseed, brewers yeast, beetroot, cabbage, carrots, clover, corn, cucumbers, green squash, olives, olive oil, papaya, peas, plums, potatoes, legumes, nuts, squash, cherries, dried dates, hummus, alfalfa sprouts, dried apricots, and mung bean sprouts.

Fatigue

Recommended supplements

- Active coenzyme form of vitamin B3
- L-carnitine
- Potassium-magnesium aspartate
- Vitamin B12
- Asian ginseng
- Fish oil
- Licorice

Best foods

- Vitamin B sources: whole grains, organ meats, sweet potatoes, avocados, egg yolks, fish, and whey. Both oatstraw and nettle infusions are good sources of B vitamins, as are red clover blossom infusion, peppermint leaves, and fenugreek seeds.
- Vitamin C sources: cantaloupe, citrus fruit and juices, kiwi, pineapple, strawberries, raspberries, broccoli, Brussel sprouts, cauliflower, green and red peppers, spinach, and tomatoes. Cooking reduces the availability of vitamin C in food. Try microwaving or steaming foods to improve availability. The best food sources of vitamin C are raw fruits and vegetables.
- Tired women need more high-quality fuel, including good fats, in their diet, especially natural sources of vitamin E, such as avocados, peanut butter, sunflower seeds, tahini, and olive oil. Herbs rich in vitamin E include nettle, seaweeds,

dandelion, and watercress.

- Celery, cabbage, seaweeds, nettle infusion, and red clover infusion are excellent sources of potassium.
- For iodine, consume seaweeds, unprocessed sea salt, mushrooms, and leafy greens grown in gardens fertilized with seaweed.
- You may need to increase your intake of iron. Consume a spoonful of molasses or take a dropperful of yellow dock tincture several times a day. Chocolate, seaweeds, red meat, liver, nettle infusions, and dandelion leaves are also superb sources of iron.
- The following foods are naturally high in vitamins and minerals and will help you sustain energy throughout the day:

   1. Peanut butter and almond butter
   2. Live-culture yoghurt
   3. Slightly underripe banana
   4. Cheese and oatcakes
   5. Turkey breast sandwich
   6. Hard-boiled egg
   7. Chicken salad on wholewheat pita bread
   8. Pasta salad
   9. Baked potato with low-fat cheese topping

I have found one of the best solutions for fatigue, apart from resting my body and mind, is to eat little and often. Breakfast is an oaty-based cereal or probiotic yoghurt with fruit. Lunch is normally Scandinavian crispbread such as Ryvita or wholemeal bread with some protein and salad, followed by pineapple (or licorice, which I'm partial to). Supper is fish or lean meat with salad or veg. Snacks include fruit mid-morning and rye bread mid-afternoon.

Vaginal Dryness

Vaginal dryness is common during and after menopause due to low estrogen, which leads to thinning of the membranes and lack of moisture. It can also mean that you are not sufficiently sexually aroused. This can occur for all sorts of reasons, such as inadequate foreplay, feelings of guilt, fear, or relationship problems.

Recommended supplements

- Acidophilus capsules inserted vaginally help prevent yeast infections and create good amounts of lubrication. Insert one or two about 4-6 hours before love making.
- Foods high in vitamin E may also help reduce dryness, or you can take a daily vitamin E supplement. Some women find that inserting a capsule of vitamin E directly into the vagina every night for a few weeks makes a difference.
- Vitamin C.

Best foods

- Boost your water intake.
- Follow a hormone-balancing diet. This includes plenty of fruit and vegetables and complex rather than simple carbohydrates, meaning whole grains like brown rice, oats, and stoneground wholemeal bread. Buy organic foods whenever possible. Eat phytoestrogen-rich foods, such as tofu, miso, soy milk, clover sprouts, flaxseed/linseed oil, and soy flour. Eat foods containing good fats, including fish, nuts, seeds, and high-quality oils, such as cold-pressed extra-virgin olive oil, and reduce your consumption of saturated fat from dairy products and red meat. Increase your daily intake of fibre. Avoid additives, preservatives, and chemicals, such as artificial sweeteners. Reduce how much caffeine you drink.

Reduce your consumption of alcohol. Avoid sugar on its own and hidden in foods.

- Natural lubricants include coconut oil, comfrey ointment, slippery elm gel, vegetable oil, aloe vera gel, raw egg white, honey, olive oil, and vitamin E oil.

WISE WOMAN WAYS

Do regular pelvic floor exercises, known as Kegel exercises. Designed to strengthen pelvic floor muscles, they also work the vagina and help to keep it healthy.

Water Retention

Recommended supplements

- Selenium

Best foods

- Foods that relieve water retention include asparagus, nettles, corn (and corn silk tea), grapes, cucumbers, watermelon (and watermelon seed tea), parsley, celery, black tea, and green tea.
- Avoid eating too much regular salt.

Strong Bones

Recommended supplements

- Calcium and magnesium
- Vitamin D
- Zinc
- Vitamin B complex
- Fish oil and EPO
- Folic acid

Best foods

- Replace bone-depleting white flour products (bread, pasta, pretzels) with fiber-rich whole grains and whole grain products.
- Eat yoghurt and fresh fruit instead of ice cream for stronger bones.
- Increase the number and amount of calcium-rich foods you consume. High levels of calcium in the diet protect you from osteoporosis, heart disease, and emotional swings. Green leafy vegetables (herbs and weeds) and milk are exceptional sources of calcium. When taking calcium supplements, ensure there is a balance of magnesium in the product.
- Cut the caffeine. It depletes calcium.
- People who drink sodas, particularly colas, may be more likely to experience bone loss and bone fractures.
- Get your soy through tofu, soy milk, soy protein, and other sources of beneficial isoflavones. For those allergic to soy, fermented soy products like tempeh and natto can often be tolerated.
- Avoid excessive salt intake and processed and restaurant foods that contain high levels of sodium, which may contribute to calcium and bone loss. Daylight, and specifically sunlight, are good sources for vitamin D.

> **WISE WOMAN WAYS**
> Gentle exercise, done regularly, helps maintain peak bone mass. Personally, if I get an urge to exercise, I lay down until it passes. However, I do enjoy gardening, daily walking, and dancing (I'm into swing and jive!).

Hot Flushes

Recommended supplements

- Isoflavones from soy or red clover.
- For hot flushes, take vitamin E daily. D-alpha tocopherol means that it comes from a natural source, but DL alpha means that it is synthetic. It may take around four weeks before the effects are really felt. Women who are diabetic, taking medication for high blood pressure, or who have rheumatic heart conditions should take vitamin E under a doctor's supervision. It's advisable that women with a history of hypertension not take high doses of vitamin E. Do not take vitamin E with digitalis.
- Royal jelly or bee pollen can reduce hot flushes for some women.
- Bioflavonoid in supplements can help relieve hot flushes.
- Asian ginseng.
- Vitamin C.
- Flavonoids.

Best foods

- Common nutritional triggers: refined carbohydrates, sugar, foods that act like sugar in the system, and simple carbohydrates, caffeine, alcohol, and hot drinks or foods (spicy or temperature-wise).
- Helpful snack foods and beverages: Non-GMO (non-genetically modified) roasted soy nuts with sea salt or other natural seasonings, raw broccoli, a bowl of oatmeal topped with three tablespoons freshly ground flax seeds and soy milk, broccoli sprouts sprinkled over a salad or tucked inside a whole-grain wrap or omelet, icy soy smoothie blended with your choice of deeply pigmented berries, iced or hot chamomile tea.

- Make foods high in phytoestrogens, such as linseed, tofu, soy milk, tempeh, and roasted soy nuts, a regular part of your diet.

Exercise helps decrease hot flushes by lowering the amount of circulating FSH and LH and by raising endorphine levels (which drop during a hot flush).

Flooding

Hormonal imbalance related to high estrogen and fluctuating progesterone, plus a sluggish liver during menopause, is the most common cause of heavy menstrual bleeding. Uterine fibroid tumours are another very common cause of excessive menstruation. Cervical polyps are small growths, the cause of which is not clear. However, they are often the result of an infection and many times associated with an abnormal response to increased estrogen levels or congestion of the blood vessels located in the cervix. Other causes of heavy menstruation include: endometrial polyps, pelvic inflammatory disease (PID), and intrauterine devices (IUDs).

Recommended supplements

- Vitamin K deficiency can cause heavy menstrual periods. If you bleed heavily but don't see a lot of clotting and you bruise easily, you could be suffering from vitamin k deficiency. It is best to get your vitamin K from foods rather than supplements. You'll find it in leafy green vegetables such as broccoli, cauliflower, spinach, and parsley.
- Vitamin E has been used to treat heavy periods. Avoid very large amounts as it can cause blood thinning.
- Essential fatty acids (EFAs) can be used to calm flooding. Take capsules or tablespoons of flaxseed oil, borage seed

oil, blackcurrant seed oil, or evening primrose oil. Borage, blackcurrant, and evening primrose oils are all high in GLA (gamma linolenic acid).

- Iron.
- Flavonoids.
- Vitamin C.
- Vitamin A.

Best foods

- If you bleed heavily, you may need extra iron to replace the iron that is being lost. Take iron in several small doses in the day rather than one large dose. Acids and proteins (orange juice or milk, for example) increase iron uptake. You may also take a liquid iron supplement, such as Floradix, during periods of heavy bleeding. For better absorption, don't drink black tea with iron supplements or meals that contain iron. Coffee, soy protein, egg yolks, bran, and calcium supplements of over 250mg impair iron absorption.
- Supplement your diet with plenty of iron-rich, dark green leafy vegetables and root vegetables, egg yolks, liver, red meat, raisins and prunes, high-quality protein, and whole grains.
- Reduce animal fats, which are converted by the body into estrogens, thus confusing feedback mechanisms. Organic, lean meats normally contain less supplemental hormones.
- Flaxseed (fresh and refrigerated to avoid the delicate oils turning rancid) can be taken in the form of flaxseed oil or by grinding refrigerated flaxseeds as you need them and sprinkling on cereal, salad, or vegetables. Consume flaxseed first thing in the morning, and drink a glass of water or herb infusion at the same time.

Avoid aspirin and specially formulated premenstrual pain relievers such as Midol, as they thin the blood (as does coumarin) and may increase bleeding. Also avoid blood-thinning herbs such as red clover, alfalfa, cleavers, pennyroyal, willow bark, and wintergreen. Thin blood is more likely to hemorrhage. Garlic can also thin the blood.

> **WISE WOMAN WAYS**
>
> I began to take serious notice of my nutrition when I was diagnosed with breast cancer many moons ago. Have to confess, though—I'm a foodie! I eat healthy food for my bowels (constipation can be an issue if I'm stressed), for my cholesterol (tad high), and for my liver (must keep the liver functioning well in order to get rid of excess hormones and toxins). I also use supplements such as bee propolis during the winter months. Happily, I occasionally fall off the good food wagon, have a ball, then get back to healthy eating. A little of what I fancy does me the world of good!

Fibroids

Uterine fibroids occur frequently in up to half of all women over 40. They are growths of smooth muscle and fibrous tissue of widely varying size in the uterus, but they may become very large. The great majority of fibroids show no symptoms, but some may cause abnormal menstrual bleeding and symptoms of pressure on the bladder that may cause you to urinate frequently.

Fibroids occur during the reproductive years when estrogen and progesterone levels are at their highest. After menopause they disappear. But because estrogen levels can rise during the early menopausal years, previously asymptomatic fibroids may grow in the years just before the cessation of menses, resulting in symptoms such as a feeling of heaviness in the belly, lower back pain, pain during vaginal penetration, urinary frequency or incontinence, bowel difficulties, or severe menstrual pain and flooding.

Recommended supplements

- Vitamin B complex
- Beta carotene
- Zinc picolinate or zinc citrate
- Vitamin E of d-alpha tocopherol
- Flaxseed oil
- Vitamin C

Best foods

- Eat organic fruit and vegetables.
- Filter your drinking water.
- Whole grains are full of lignins (compounds that have an antiestrogenic effect on the body). Eat plenty of rye, millet, soy products (especially fermented soy products such as miso and tempeh), oats, buckwheat, barley, corn, and brown rice.
- Have two tablespoons of cracked linseed each day (in soups, salads, stir fry, or on baked potatoes).
- Reduce your intake of animal fats. Essential fats found in nuts and seeds are fine.
- A good guideline is to eat 50 percent of your foods in their raw state each day.
- Avoid coffee, cocoa, flour products, dairy, chocolate, and sugar, and stay away from cheap, junk fats, margarine, and golden cooking oil.
- Make sure that vegetables are thoroughly washed with apple cider vinegar or lemon juice to help remove the pesticides,

as these affect the body much like synthetic estrogen. Ideally, use organic vegetables that are untreated with pesticides.

- Make sure you eat a high-fibre diet.
- Limit meat to three times a week. Cheaply produced meat and dairy products from animals raised in crowded, unsanitary conditions on large feedlots contain significant amounts of estrogen from being treated with hormones to speed up animal growth. With high-quality proteins such as organic meat and dairy, free-range eggs, and wild-caught fish, you don't need to eat as much in order to feel satisfied, and you will be nutritionally better off as they contain fewer or no added hormones. Vegetable protein sources contain beneficial complex carbohydrates and are less acid forming than meat.
- High-quality protein foods that have a good balance of amino acids include eggs, quinoa (an ancient grain that cooks like rice), seed veg (runner beans, peas, corn, broccoli), cottage cheese, nuts and seeds, soy (tofu), organic meat and fish, and beans and lentils.

Where there is estrogen dominance in the body, progesterone balances out the excess. When enough progesterone is supplied, fibroid growth is arrested. Other solutions for balancing out estrogen include:

- Decrease stress. When you take in a stimulant, such as coffee, or react stressfully to an event, the body produces the essential adrenal hormone cortisol. This hormone competes with progesterone for receptor sites (sites within the body that would normally receive progesterone to balance out the estrogen). As a result, the effect of being in an ongoing stressed state is less active progesterone in the body.

Cortisol also increases production of estrogen, so prolonged stress can contribute to estrogen dominance.

- Normally, the liver can easily deal with slight excesses of estrogen, but if your diet is poor, you suffer from allergies, or take in excessive toxins, your liver's ability to detoxify and eliminate estrogen can be impaired (a herbal detox may be a good idea).
- Increase nutrients in the diet. Follow a hormone-balancing diet consisting of lots of fresh fruits and vegetables, adequate protein, complex carbohydrates—such as whole grains—and moderate amounts of healthy fat. Block excess estrogen with phytoestrogenic foods such as flaxseed and soy.
- Apply topical bioidentical progesterone cream to block the effects of overproduction of estrogen.
- Lose excess body fat and get regular exercise, especially strength training.

WISE WOMAN WAYS

Fibroids, suggests Dr Christiane Northrup[15] are symbolic of creativity waiting to be birthed. They may also result when we are putting our life force into relationships (personal or professional) that have no meaning for us. Consider:

- What creations within me do I wish to bring into existence?
- If I could have or be anything, how would I choose to live my life?
- If I had six months to live, who would I choose to be with for nourishment and inspiration?

The Menopause Healthy Eating Plan

Ensure your vegetables, salad greens, fruit, and meats are as organic as you can afford. Drink at least 2 litres of water a day. Limit your intake of red meat, processed foods, salt (whether added or in cooking), and alcohol. Tea and coffee should be replaced by caffeine-free drinks.

You may want to add to your diet soy-based foods such as tofu and soy milk, particularly emphasizing fermented soy products such as miso and tempeh; legumes (chickpeas, beans, and so on); bean sprouts; yams; most fruit and vegetables, particularly celery and rhubarb; and almonds and linseeds. All of these foods contain healthful phytoestrogens (plants with weak estrogenlike effects in the body).

You should also keep your intake of calcium food high, so that your bones remain strong; weakening is more likely during menopause as estrogen levels drop. Drink semi-skimmed or skimmed milk. Other good calcium sources include almonds, seeds (poppy, sesame), cheeses (Parmesan is easy to digest and high in protein, or Gruyère and Edam), oily coldwater fish (tinned sardines, salmon, and so on), tofu, seaweed if you're a fan of Japanese food, figs, yoghurt, Brazil nuts, and leafy vegetables, such as kale and purple broccoli.

Limit your wheat intake to only two slices of granary or whole grain bread a day. I advise limiting wheat and the gluten it contains, because an excess can cause weight gain, blood sugar imbalances (leading to energy crashes), and bloating.

To keep your blood sugar levels balanced and avoid fatigue, spread your food intake and, ideally, consume five small meals a day—breakfast, lunch, and dinner, plus a mid-morning and mid-afternoon snack. Ensure you have protein with each sitting:

Breakfast
- Porridge or other oat-based cereal
- Egg on toast
- Yoghurt with seeds

Mid-morning snack	• Small handful of unsalted nuts and fruit
Lunch	• If you didn't have bread at breakfast, a sandwich with lean ham, cheese, oily fish, hummus, or egg, accompanied by a salad, with fruits such as berries or yoghurt for dessert
	• Baked potato with cheese, oily fish, hummus, or egg, followed by fruit or yoghurt
	• Salad of legumes, with fruit or yoghurt for dessert
	• Soup made from lentils or other legumes, with fruit or yoghurt for dessert
	• Oatcakes, Scandinavian crispbread like Ryvita, or rice cakes with lean ham, cheese, oily fish, paté, or egg salad, with fruit or yoghurt for dessert
	• Lean ham, cheese, tofu, oily fish, or egg, accompanied by salad and with fruit or yoghurt for dessert.
Mid-afternoon snack	• Small handful of unsalted nuts and fruit
Dinner	• Chicken, tofu, a meat substitute like quorn, lean red meat, or oily fish with salad
	• Chicken, tofu, quorn, lean red meat, or oily fish with vegetables.

An additional tip given to me by my grandmother is to start the day off with a cup of hot water and lemon juice. It kick-starts the liver and does wonders for the skin.

> **WISE WOMAN WAYS**
> Seaweeds of all kinds help restore energy by nourishing the nervous, immune, and hormonal systems. Make it a habit to eat seaweed as a green vegetable at least once a week. Try kelp in your oatmeal, wakame in your beans, kombu in your soups, hijiki salads, toasted dulse, sea palm fronds, and deep-fried nori and sushi.

What Happens Next?

A nourishing diet during our menopause years will help our bodies ease through the Change. As Wise Women, we also know the value of using herbs as part of our daily nutrition. I cover this in the chapter that follows.

Useful Resources

Organizations

- British Association for Applied Nutrition and Nutritional Therapy, *www.bant.org.uk* (for listings of qualified nutritional therapists)
- American Dietetic Association, *www.eatright.org* (for registered dieticians)

Supplements

- The Nutri Centre, *www.nutricentre.com*

CHAPTER 4

Wort Cunning

The Wise Woman going through her menopause years will embrace the use of herbs (ideally organic) into her healing regime.

Liver

- DANDELION has been used for many years as a general liver tonic, making it a useful menopause herb in an indirect way. The liver filters all that we eat and drink, as well as medications, toxins, and hormones. When a women's hormone production level becomes unbalanced, the liver undergoes a great deal of stress.
- MILK THISTLE strengthens the liver.
- YELLOW DOCK ROOT helps to metabolize estrogen out of the body, thus reducing fibroids.

Low Libido

- DAMIANA is a herb that is frequently used to stimulate the female libido.
- SARSAPARILLA is a herb that stimulates the production of testosterone and therefore improves a waning libido.
- OATSTRAW can be consumed in the form of oats for breakfast, an excellent way to take this herb into your body.
- MACA ROOT has been used for centuries in South America and is an adaptogen, meaning it helps to balance the body's hormonal system as needed.

Bladder

- SAW PALMETTO is available as a dried fruit extract and is an astringent diuretic herb that can treat urinary incontinence, fluid retention, and prolapse of the pelvic organs. It will also reduce the dryness and lack of tone in the tissues of the bladder which so often lead to irritation and weakness. Many women use it to combat chronic urinary tract infections.

Bone Strength

- YAMS are a powerful estrogenic food that can provide relief by acting as an anti-inflammatory agent to alleviate menopausal arthritis.
- OATSTRAW as an infusion keeps the bones strong.
- NETTLE protects bones.
- RED CLOVER is one of the premium sources of phytoestrogens. It contains high amounts of calcium and may slow down bone loss.
- MACA ROOT contains high levels of calcium, magnesium, zinc, and iron, as well as vitamins B1, B2, B12, C, and E.

WISE WOMAN WAYS

Herbal sources of phytoestrogens include ginseng, horsetail, black cohosh, dong quai, and licorice root, hops, sage, red clover, agnus castus, fennel, wild yam, bladderwrack, and sarsparilla. NOTE: Some women need to be cautious of taking herbal supplements if they have breast cancer or other hormone-dependent tumours.

Heavy Bleeding

- WILD YAM (progestogenic properties)
- AGRIMONY
- CRAMP BARK and VALERIAN (and cramps)
- LADY'S MANTLE (and cramps).
- BIOFLAVONOIDS strengthen capillaries and provide estrogenic factors that help decrease flooding. Plants containing bioflavonoids include dong quai, black cohosh, blue cohosh, unicorn root, false unicorn root, fennel, anise, sarsparilla, and wild yam root. Generally, yellow, orange, and red vegetables and fruits are good sources of bioflavonoids.
- RASPBERRY LEAF is a nutritive estrogenic herb and astringent that works directly on the uterus, toning weakened muscles and relaxing uterine spasms.
- SAGE (blood clots in heavy bleed).
- SHEPHERDS PURSE (often taken with yarrow) functions as a pituitary regulator with androgenic properties to normalize progesterone levels.
- STINGING NETTLE.
- AGNUS CASTUS helps the body produce progesterone, which balances estrogen (takes a couple of cycles to kick in and needs to be taken daily).
- CINNAMON BARK relieves uterine cramping and checks flooding.
- DANDELION LEAVES and YELLOW DOCK ROOT are excellent for flooding as they contain a bioavailable form of iron, which is lost in excessive flooding.
- WITCH HAZEL allows normal menstruation and has a tonic effect on the uterus.

Fibroids

- MISTLETOE and BUTTERBUR are good in combination for use in shrinking fibroids.

WISE WOMAN WAYS

A herbal tea, or tisane, is a (hot or cold) herbal infusion made from the combination of boiling water and fresh or dried flowers, leaves, seeds, or roots. The tisane is then strained before drinking. The longer the infusion steeps, the stronger the qualities of the herb you drink.

I'm having some flooding at the moment. In speaking to my homeopath, we discussed the differences between making herbal tea or taking a herbal tincture. The outcome of the conversation was that there's not much difference between the two. However, making fresh herbal tea with dried herbs is much better than herbal tea bags.

I've chosen to drink a tea made up of a combination of ladies mantle and raspberry leaf (two heaped teaspoons into a teapot and infused for 10 minutes). I drink this once a day normally—three times a day when I'm bleeding. The tea tastes good, and I like the ritual of making this tea and sitting quietly to drink it.

Here are some common herbs you might like to experiment with: catnip (calming), dill (upset stomach), fennel (weight loss), chamomile (calming), ginseng (stimulating), hibiscus (consumed in Okinawa, where the natives associate it with longevity), rosemary (memory), and purple sage (calming).

Vaginal Dryness

- DONG QUAI, BLACK COHOSH, and SLIPPERY ELM can be spread inside the vulva and vagina. Mix two tablespoons of the powder in a cup of water and heat, stirring until thick. Be sure to cool before use.
- CHICKWEED.
- COMFREY OINTMENT can be rubbed in morning and night and used as a lubricant for love making.
- ALOE GEL: Put directly on the vagina to soothe dryness and irritation.
- MOTHERWORT and AGNUS CASTUS are thought to regulate hormones and may help restore thickness and elasticity to the vagina.
- MACA ROOT helps balance out our body's hormone system.

Water Retention

- DANDELION strengthens the liver and helps it process excess hormones.
- CLEAVERS herb tincture tells the lymphatic tissues to get moving and is especially helpful for swollen, sore breasts.
- EVENING PRIMROSE OIL is an adaptogen and useful for fluid retention.

Headaches

Chinese herbalists say headaches are caused by liver stress. Liver-strengthening herbs are dandelion, yellow dock, milk thistle seed, and burdock.

- SAGE offers relief from headaches.
- SOY is a phytoestrogen and can help with migraine headaches.

- SKULLCAP can ease pain and relieve muscle spasms.
- EVENING PRIMROSE OIL is an adaptogen and useful for headaches.

Dry Eyes

- OATSTRAW infusion cools and moistens your eyes from the inside out.
- CHAMOMILE tea bags soaked in mildly warm or cool water.
- FRESH CHICKWEED applied as a poultice to the closed eyes will help.

Hot Flushes

- EVENING PRIMROSE OIL alleviates hot flushes and promotes restful sleep.
- CHICKWEED tincture reduces the severity and frequency of hot flushes.
- GINSENG (American or Korean) capsules. Ginseng works best on an empty stomach and can be taken before breakfast and before dinner. It is recommended that you not eat fruit for two hours after taking ginseng and that you take it separately from any vitamin supplement. It is not advised for women with high blood pressure or diabetes. Women with asthma or emphysema would do well to avoid ginseng because of its histamine-liberating properties.
- BIOFLAVONOIDS are very effective in controlling hot flushes, anxiety, and irritability. Plants containing bioflavonoids include dong quai, black cohosh, blue cohosh, unicorn root, false unicorn root, fennel, anise, sarsparilla, and wild yam root. Generally, yellow, orange, and red vegetables and fruits are good sources of bioflavonoids.

- Many women experience relief from hot flushes with the topical use of a bioidentical progesterone cream made from extract of wild Mexican yam.
- NETTLE can help prevent night sweats.
- RED CLOVER is one of the premium sources of phytoestrogens, weak plant estrogens that help increase levels of estrogen in our bodies, thereby reducing menopausal symptoms. Red clover also contains many vitamins and minerals, including calcium, magnesium, niacin, potassium, and vitamin C.
- DANDELION is a superb strengthener for the liver, the control center for hot flushes.
- SAGE appears to be especially useful for the treatment of hot flushes, as it contains plant estrogens.
- BLACK COHOSH is a phytoestrogen and has been shown to control hot flushes by reducing the effects of the lutenizing hormone in the body.
- DONG QUAI is a herb native to China. It is known as the "female ginseng" and is viewed as one of the foremost herbs in treating symptoms of menopause. It contains phytoestrogens that bind to the estrogen receptors in the body, thereby increasing levels of estrogen. In particular, dong quai dilates the blood vessels, thereby increasing blood flow and helping to relieve hot flushes. Dong quai is especially effective when used in combination with black cohosh.
- MACA ROOT is an adaptogen and benefits the hypothalamus and pituitary, both of which are part of the adrenal system. Hot flushes are caused by wrong signals to the body from the hypothalamus, responsible for regulating body heat.
- MOTHERWORT is great for hot flushes and night sweats, but it also regulates blood pressure and the adrenal system.

Mood Swings

- EVENING PRIMROSE OIL is an adaptogen and useful for mood swings, anxiety, and irritability.
- SOY is a phytoestrogen and can help with mood swings.
- LICORICE ROOT is a phytoestrogen and can help with mood swings and menopausal depression due to its activity on specific neurotransmitters.
- OATSTRAW strengthens the nerves, helps reduce emotion distress.
- DAMIANA can act as a mild antidepressant.
- NETTLE will strengthen the adrenals and ease anxiety.
- TRUE UNICORN ROOT is an estrogenic herb and provides a mild sedative action.
- ASHWAGANDHA is an adaptogen and is used as a herb for gentle relaxation and emotional balance.
- RED CLOVER grows naturally in Europe and Asia and is one of the premium sources of phytoestrogens, the weak plant estrogens that help increase estrogen levels in the body, thereby reducing menopausal symptoms. Studies on red clover show that it does seem to reduce symptoms of mood swings in menopause.
- AGNUS CASTUS is useful as a menopause herb as it alleviates the symptoms of depression.
- MOTHERWORT has a calming effect but does not make you drowsy.
- BLACK COHOSH is touted as a great reliever of anxiety and depression. Black cohosh may be taken up to twice a day for six months, but should not be taken for a longer period of time.
- DONG QUAI is nicknamed the "female ginseng" and contains phytoestrogens. Dong quai is a mild sedative that will

help reduce mood swings and stress related to menopause. Dong quai is especially effective when used in combination with black cohosh.

WISE WOMAN WAYS

My garden is large and rural, although I live on the outskirts of a large city. I leave the beds to do their own thing (with a little pruning), and there are loads of plants in pots everywhere. I would love to grow herbs but don't, for two reasons. One is the slugs and snails that insist on taking their package holidays throughout the year with us. Secondly, I get through the herbs too fast. So I have to confess to doing the modern Wise Woman thing and getting my fresh culinary herbs from our local organic greengrocer up the road, my medicinal tinctures from an organic herbalist, and my fresh dried herbs for tea from Neal's Yard in Covent Garden, London.

Insomnia

- OATSTRAW in the form of a tincture promotes sound sleep. An excellent way of getting this herb through the diet is to eat oats for breakfast.

Fatigue

- OATSTRAW infusion builds energy and eases anxiety.
- NETTLE INFUSION increases energy without wiring your nerves. Nettle strengthens the adrenals, allowing you to tolerate more stress with less harm. The plants with the deepest green give you the most energy. Drink a daily cup of nettle infusion for fatigue.

- GINSENG strengthens the adrenal glands, increases immunity, boosts energy, and normalizes blood pressure. It can be used for treating mental and physical fatigue. Siberian ginseng has been shown to be somewhat more effective than the American variety. Asian ginseng is an adaptogen and helps the body resist stress and adapt to change.
- SARSPARILLA can increase energy and overall feelings of vitality.
- LICORICE acts as a powerful adrenal stimulant and estrogenic herb. The effect on the adrenal gland is enhanced by adding Asian ginseng. It also blocks the activity of a specific enzyme that subsequently increases the activity of cortisol (helpful for adrenal fatigue). Note: if you have high blood pressure, you need to be careful about the stimulating effect of licorice; however, if you have low blood pressure, licorice could be beneficial.

Healthy Heart

- RED CLOVER is one of the premium sources of phytoestrogens. Red clover increases the amount of high-density lipoprotein (HDL), or "good" cholesterol, in the bloodstream. An excellent way of getting this herb through the diet is to eat oats as an early evening snack. Higher levels of HDL have been linked to a reduction in the risk of heart disease in menopausal women.

Circulation

- GINKGO improves brain function, circulation, and oxygenation of all body cells. This action relieves symptoms of depression, fatigue, and the memory problems associated with the transition into menopause.

Herbal Sources of Vitamins

- VITAMIN B COMPLEX: For healthy digestion, good liver function, emotional flexibility, less anxiety, sound sleep, milder hot flushes, and steady heart beat. Depleted by hormone replacement treatment (HRT). *Herbal sources:* Red clover blossoms, parsley leaf, and oatstraw.

- VITAMIN B1 (thiamine): For emotional ease, strong nerves. *Herbal sources:* Peppermint, burdock, sage, yellow dock, alfalfa, red clover, fenugreek seeds, raspberry leaves, nettle, catnip, watercress, yarrow leaf/flower, and rose buds and hips.

- VITAMIN B2 (riboflavin): For more energy, healthy skin. Depleted by: hot flushes. *Herbal sources:* Peppermint, alfalfa greens, parsley, echinacea, yellow dock, hops, dandelion root, ginseng, dulse, kelp, fenugreek seed, rose hips, and nettles.

- VITAMIN B9 (folic acid): For strong, flexible bones and calm nerves. *Herbal sources:* Leafy greens of nettles, alfalfa, parsley, sage, catnip, peppermint, plantain, comfrey, and chickweed.

- VITAMIN B3 (niacin): For relief of anxiety and depression, decrease in headaches, and reduction of serum cholesterol levels. *Herbal sources:* Hops, raspberry leaf, red clover; slippery elm, echinacea, licorice, rose hips, nettle, alfalfa, and parsley.

- BIOFLAVONOIDS: For a healthy heart and to reduce hot flushes and night sweats, menstrual bleeding, breast lumps, water retention, and anxiety. *Herbal sources:* Buckwheat greens, elderberries, hawthorn fruits, rose hips, horsetail, shepherd's purse, and chervil.

- CAROTENES: For a well-lubricated vagina, strong bones, protection against cancer, and healthy lungs and skin.

Herbal sources: Peppermint, yellow dock, uva ursi, parsley, alfalfa, raspberry, nettles, dandelion greens, kelp, green onions, violet leaves, cayenne, paprika, lamb's quarters leaves, sage, chickweed, horsetail, black cohosh roots, and rose hips.

- VITAMIN C COMPLEX: For less intense hot flushes, insomnia, and night sweats, stronger bones, fewer headaches, better resistance to infection, and easier emotions. Critical to good adrenal functioning, especially during menopause. Depleted by stress and aging. *Herbal sources:* Rose hips, yellow dock root, raspberry leaf, red clover, hops, pine needles, dandelion greens, alfalfa greens, echinacea, skullcap, plantain, parsley, cayenne, and paprika.

- VITAMIN E: for milder hot flushes, fewer night sweats, protection from cancer, fewer signs of aging, fewer wrinkles, moist vagina, strong heart, and freedom from arthritis. Depleted by hormone replacement therapy (HRT). *Herbal sources:* Alfalfa, rosehips, nettles, dong quai, watercress, dandelion, seaweeds, and wild seeds of lamb's quarters and plantain.

- ESSENTIAL FATTY ACIDS (EFAS), including GLA, OMEGA-6, and OMEGA-3: For a healthy heart, less severe hot flushes, strong nerves, strong bones, well-functioning endocrine glands, and fewer wrinkles. All wild plants, but very few cultivated plants, contain EFAs; fresh purslane is notably high.

- VITAMIN K: For less menstrual flooding and stronger bones. *Herbal sources:* Nettle, alfalfa, kelp, green tea.

WISE WOMAN WAYS

Herbal honeys are made by pouring honey over fresh herbs and allowing them to infuse over a period of several days to several months. As the herbs are infused with honey, the water-loving honey absorbs all the water-soluble and anti-infective volatile oils of the herb. Here's how to create your herbal honey:

- Coarsely chop the dried herb of your choice (ginger and garlic should be used fresh). You could use sage, rose, mint, oregano, lemon vervena, lavender, fennel seeds, thyme, rosemary, marjoram, or lemon balm.
- Put chopped herb into a wide-mouthed jar, filling almost to the top.
- Pour pasteurized honey into the jar, working it into the herb with a wooden spoon.
- Fill the jar to the very top and cover tightly and label.

Your herbal honey is ready to use in as little as a day or two, but will be more medicinal if allowed to sit for six weeks. Ways to use your herbal honey include spreading it on homemade bread, placing a tablespoonful (include herb as well as honey) into a mug of boiling water, eating by the spoonful right from the jar to soothe and heal sore throats, or smearing the honey minus herb onto wounds and burns.

Herbal Sources of Minerals

- BORON: For strong, flexible bones. *Herbal sources:* All organic garden weeds, including all edible parts of chickweed, purslane, nettles, dandelion, and yellow dock.

- CALCIUM: For sound sleep, dense bones, freedom from depression and headaches, less bloating, and fewer mood fluctuations. *Herbal sources:* Valerian, kelp, nettle, horsetail, peppermint; sage, uva ursi, yellow dock, chickweed, red clover, oatstraw, parsley, black currant leaf, raspberry leaf, plantain leaf/seed, dandelion leaf, amaranth leaf/seed, and lamb's quarter leaf/seed.

- CHROMIUM: For less fatigue, fewer mood swings, stable blood sugar levels, and increased high-density lipoprotein (HDL), known as the "good" cholesterol. *Herbal sources:* Oatstraw, nettle, red clover tops, catnip, dulse, wild yam, yarrow, horsetail; roots of black cohosh, licorice, echinacea, valerian, and sarsparilla.

- COPPER: For supple skin, healthy hair, calm nerves, less water retention, less menstrual flooding, and lower serum cholesterol. *Herbal sources:* Skullcap, sage, horsetail, and chickweed.

- IODINE: For fewer breast lumps, less fatigue, and stronger liver. *Herbal sources:* Kelp, parsley, celery, and sarsparilla root.

- IRON: For fewer hot flushes and headaches, less menstrual flooding, better sleep with fewer night sweats, calmer nerves, more energy, and less dizziness. *Herbal sources:* Chickweed, kelp, burdock root, catnip, horsetail, Althea root, milk thistle seed, uva ursi, dandelion leaf/root; yellow dock, dong quai, black cohosh, echinacea, licorice, valerian, and sarsparilla roots; and nettles, plantain leaf, fenugreek seed, and peppermint.

- MAGNESIUM: For deeper sleep, less anxiety, easier nerves, flexible bones, lower low-density lipoprotein (LDL), or "bad," cholesterol, more energy, and fewer headaches/migraines. Depleted by hot flushes and night sweats. *Herbal sources:* Oatstraw, licorice, kelp, nettle, dulse, burdock root, chickweed, Althea root, horsetail, sage, raspberry leaf, red clover, valerian, yellow dock, dandelion greens, carrot tops, parsley leaf, evening primrose.

- MANGANESE: For flexible bones and a reduction in dizziness. *Herbal sources:* Raspberry, uva ursi leaf, chickweed, milk thistle seed, yellow dock; ginseng, wild yam, echinacea, and dandelion roots; and nettle, catnip, kelp, horsetail, and hops flowers.

- MOLYBDENUM: For fewer hot flushes and prevention of anemia. *Herbal sources:* Nettles, dandelion greens, sage, oatstraw, fenugreek seeds, raspberry leaves, red clover blossoms, horsetail, chickweed, and kelp.

- NICKEL: For milder hot flushes and calmer nerves. *Herbal sources:* Alfalfa, red clover, oatstraw, and fenugreek.

- PHOSPHORUS: For strong, flexible bones, more energy. *Herbal sources:* Peppermint, yellow dock, milk thistle, fennel, hops, chickweed, nettle, dandelion, parsley, dulse, and red clover.

- POTASSIUM: For more energy, less fatigue, less water retention, easy weight loss, steady heart beat, and better digestion. Depleted by hot flushes and night sweats. *Herbal sources:* Sage, catnip, peppermint, skullcap, hops, dulse, kelp, red clover, horsetail, nettles, and plantain leaf.

- SELENIUM: For slower aging, strong immunity, less irritability, more energy, healthy hair/nails/teeth, and less cardiovascular disease. *Herbal sources:* Catnip, milk thistle seed, valerian root, dulse, black cohosh and ginseng roots; uva ursi leaf, hops flowers, kelp, raspberry leaf, rose buds and hips, hawthorn berries, fenugreek seed, roots of echinacea, sarsparilla, and yellow dock.

- SILICON: For strong, flexible bones, less irritable nerves. *Herbal sources:* Horsetail, dulse, echinacea, cornsilk, burdock, oatstraw, licorice, chickweed, uva ursi, and sarsparilla.
- SULFUR: For soft skin and glossy hair, healthy nerves, and strong liver. *Herbal sources:* Sage, nettles, plantain, and horsetail.
- ZINC: For slower aging, better digestion, stronger bones, healthy skin, cancer prevention, and increased sex drive. Depleted by hormone replacement therapy (HRT). *Herbal sources:* Skullcap, sage, wild yam, chickweed, echinacea, nettles, dulse, milk thistle, and sarsparilla.

WISE WOMAN WAYS

If you are on ANY medication, please consult a qualified medical herbalist[16] before taking herbs as there can be distressing interactions between some pharmaceutical medications and herbal compounds.

What Happens Next?

The use of herbs in Wise Woman healing, both internally and externally, is part of our sacred heritage. While flower essences aren't to be confused with herbs or essential oils, they too have their precious place in our life during the menopause years. Read on to discover how you might use these gifts from nature.

CHAPTER 5

Using Flower Essences During Menopause

From the beginning of time, nature has provided the means to heal on all levels. Flower essences have been used for centuries in Australia, South America, Asia, Egypt, South America, and India. They were also very popular in Europe in the Middle Ages. Hildegard von Bingen, a 12th-century visionary who wrote medicinal texts, and Paracelsus, a 15th-century physician and astrologer, both wrote how they used dew collected from flowering plants to treat health imbalances.

How Flower Essences Work

Flower essences are a form of vibrational medicine and act in a similar way to homeopathic remedies by working with subtle energy in the body. All living things, including our body and mind, are matter that is permeated and surrounded by, subtle energy. We could define subtle energy as the underpinning source feeding the well-being of our mind and body.

According to the concept of energy medicine, disease manifests in the physical body only after energy flow in the subtle body has been disturbed. Energy medicine has been long been practiced by civilizations such as India and China, and is gradually being integrated into Western healthcare. The energy field model used by these civilizations as part of their eclectic healthcare system, which includes acupuncture, moves away from the singular idea that life evolves from a scientific blueprint, towards the concept that life circulates via electrical charges of energy known as *prana* or *chi*. In addition to this circulation of energy, there is a force field of energy permeating the human body called the aura, which can influence our well-being. In order to rebalance the subtle body, we must administer energy that vibrates at frequencies beyond the physical plane. Just as we might heal the physical body through medical interventions, we need to heal the subtle body through vibrational interventions such as homeopathy, crystals, or flower essences.

Flower essences work by utilizing the essence's positive energy to transmute a negative state in living things, whether they be human, animal, or plant. Each flower used in a flower essence conveys a subtle energy pattern that is transferred to water during essence preparation. This preparation is then either used internally or externally for healing purposes.

From a spiritual perspective, flower essences address mental and emotional imbalances that, if left unresolved, could influence the wellness of the physical body. In effect, we "co-create" with the flower essences to alter our subtle energies when we use them for healing purposes. This change permeates our emotional and mental states and can also influence our physical well-being. The belief that we can heal ourselves is the basis of flower essence philosophy.

Essences do not affect us biochemically, as does traditional allopathic medicine. They are water-based products that have no chemical or biological materials present other than water and alcohol preservatives such as brandy, vodka, and so on.

Bach Flower Remedies

Dr Edward Bach[17] studied medicine at University College Hospital, London, qualified in 1912, and became casualty medical officer at the hospital in 1913. He worked in general practice in London's famed medical sector Harley Street and as a bacteriologist and pathologist working on vaccines. In the course of his work, he came to question some of the tenets of early 20th-century medical practice. Bach believed that the illness-personality link was a product of unbalanced energetic patterns within the subtle body, and that illness was a reflection of disharmony between the physical personality and the Higher Self.

Bach took a post at the Royal London Homeopathic Hospital (1919), where he noticed the parallels between his work on vaccines and the principles of homoeopathy. Although his work up to this point had been with bacteria, he wanted to find healing modalities that would be less toxic and more in tune with the mind-body link. To this end, he began collecting plants in the hope of replacing the nosodes (homeopathic remedies prepared from infected tissues) with a series of gentler remedies.

In 1928, Bach acquired two wildflowers, impatiens and mimulus, which he homeopathically prepared and clinically used with excellent results. He soon understood that there was great healing power in flowers, and he gradually developed his own methods of preparing flower essences. In the early 1930s, Bach left his successful practice and began gathering wildflowers, which he developed into 38 flower remedies.

Instead of scientific methodology, he chose to rely on his intuitive gifts as a healer. He found that he could place the flowers of a particular species on the surface of a bowl of springwater for several hours in sunlight and obtain powerful vibrational tinctures. The subtle effects of sunlight charged the water with an energetic imprint of the flower's unique signature.

In 1934, Dr Bach moved to Mount Vernon in Oxfordshire, England, and it was here, in the surrounding countryside, that he found the remaining flower remedies he sought, each aimed at a particular mental state or emotion. Significantly, Bach's work was in tune with nature's own annual cycle. In spring and summer, he found the flowers he needed in the countryside and prepared individual flower remedies, then in winter, he helped and advised patients. He found that when he treated the feelings of his patients, their distress and physical discomfort would be alleviated to allow their natural healing to come through.

The 38 Bach Flower Remedies include:

agrimony	aspen
beech	centaury
cerato	cherry plum
chestnut bud	chicory
clematis	crab apple
elm	gentian
gorse	heather
holly	honeysuckle
hornbeam	impatiens
larch	mimulus
mustard	oak
olive	pine
red chestnut	rock rose
rock water	schleranthus
star of Bethlehem	sweet chestnut
vervain	vine
walnut	water violet
white chestnut	wild oat
wild rose	willow

Menopausal State	Recommended Bach Flower Remedy
Apprehensive, anxious	aspen, larch, mimulus
Depression	cherry plum, gentian, gorse, mustard, white chestnut, and wild rose
Dissatisfaction	wild oat
Fretful	agrimony

Fuzzy thinking, lack of concentration	crab apple, clematis
Hot flushes	cherry plum, impatiens, larch, mimulus, and walnut
Indecisive, self-doubting	cerato, scleranthus, wild oat
Insomnia	holly, hornbeam, mustard, olive, white chestnut
Intolerant, critical, irritable	beech, holly, impatiens, rock water, vervain, vine
Irrational without knowing why	cherry plum
Lack of confidence	centaury, larch, and mimulus
Lack of sexual interest	clematis
Managing change	walnut
Nit-picking over detail	crab apple
Overburdened	hornbeam, olive
Overwhelmed	elm
Panic	cherry plum, rock rose
Procrastination	hornbeam
Prone to making mistakes	chestnut bud
Resentful	willow
Sadness, loss (of youth)	star of Bethlehem
Sudden anger	
Uncomfortable/	beech, cherry plum, holly, rock water
ashamed with body	crab apple
Tired, drained	olive

I came to the Bach Flower Remedies about 25 years ago. A friend had a computer and photocopy shop and I would sometimes help out. One day a nutritionist came in with a mound of copying to do, much of it related to flower essences. Being full of curiosity, I was reading as I was copying. It was like coming home. I learnt the remedies by using them on myself, and since those days all the remedies have been in my home ready to use with family, friends, animals, plants, clients, students, and myself.

Animals and young children respond particularly well to Bach Flower Remedies. I remember going to an animal sanctuary on the request of a student of mine who worked there. In a glass terrarium were a mother snake and several babies. Mum snake, bless her, had a cold and was coiled in a corner. I made up a remedy for the student to give to the mother snake, and within minutes she picked up and got right into a bit of family entwining! I've given remedies to cats following operations and dogs in crisis over fireworks night. I've also had lots of success giving remedies to babies and young children with sleep and behavioural issues at the parent's request. I've found that it's important to use the remedy or remedies that resonate as the right ones at the gut level—however off the wall they might seem at the time. It's a good idea to carry Bach Flower Rescue Remedy as an emergency stress-buster. It's a mixture of rock rose, impatiens, clematis, star of Bethlehem, and cherry plum and works rapidly to calm the body.

Australian Bush Flower Essences

Since Dr. Bach created his flower essences in the 1930s, the issues we face in our lives have changed. As we came to the end of the 20th century and slipped into the 21st century, there was a growing need for flower essences that help people deal with the issues of today.

While many new flower essences have found their way to the commercial market, some of the most effective new flower essences come from Australian plants [18] as a result of the work of Ian White, a naturopath and fifth-generation Australian herbalist. Ian grew up in the Australian bush. As a young boy his grandmother, like her mother before her, specialized in using Australian plants and would often take him bush walking to learn the healing qualities of plants and flowers. He learned a profound respect for nature through her and went on to become a practitioner and a pioneer working with and researching the rare remedial qualities of Australian native plants. Australia is relatively unpolluted, has some of the world's oldest plants, and metaphysically has a wise, old energy.

The 65 Australian Bush Essences include:

alpine mint bush	angelsword
banksia robur	bauhinia
billy goat plum	black-eyed Susan
bluebell	boab
boronia	bottlebrush
bush fuchsia	bush gardenia
bush iris	crowea
dagger hakea	dog rose
dog rose of wild forces	five corners
flannel flower	freshwater mangrove
fringed violet	green spider orchid
grey spider flower	gymea lily
hibbertia	illawarra flame tree
isopogon	jacaranda
kangaroo paw	kapok bush
little flannel flower	macrocarpa
mint bush	mountain devil
mulla mulla	old man banksia
paw paw	peach-flowered tea tree
philotheca	pink mulla mulla
red grevillea	red helmet orchid
red lily	red suva frangipani
rough bluebell	she oak

silver princess
Southern Cross
sturt desert pea
sundew
tall mulla mulla
turkey bush
wedding bush
wisteria

slender rice flower
spinifex
sturt desert rose
sunshine wattle
tall yellow top
waratah
wild potato bush
yellow cowslip orchid

Menopausal State	Recommended Australian Bush Essence
Apprehensive, anxious	tall mulla mulla, dog rose, illawarra flame tree
Constipation	bauhinia, bottlebrush, flannel flower, bluebell
Creative block	turkey bush, bush fuchsia
Depression	waratah, tall yellow top
Fear of intimacy	flannel flower
Hormone imbalance	she oak
Hot flushes	mulla mulla
Indecisive, self-doubting	five corners, kapok bush, red grevillea
Insomnia	boronia, grey spider flower, black-eyed Susan, and crowea
Intolerant, critical, irritable	yellow cowslip orchid, mountain devil, and black-eyed Susan
Lack of confidence	five corners, kapok bush
Lack of sexual interest	billy goat plum
Managing change	bauhinia, bottlebrush, mint bush, pink
mulla mulla,	and silver princess
Mental and	
emotional exhaustion	alpine mint bush, banksia robur, macrocarpa

Palpitations	waratah, jacaranda, crowea, bush fuchsia, and bluebell
Panic	grey spider flower, dog rose of the wild forces
Resentful	dagger hakea
Sadness, loss (of youth)	peach-flowered tea tree
Uncomfortable/ ashamed of body	billy goat plum, wild potato bush, wisteria, spinifex
Tired, drained	old man banksia
Worry	crowea

The Australian Bush Essences found me through a book—or rather that's how I remembered them again. While I have never been to Australia, there is some link to this wild country in my soul. I've used these essences increasingly over the years and find them very profound in their action.

Combination Mixtures

While you can be purist and use just the Bach Flower Remedies or the Australian Bush Essences, you can also mix the two together. Using a blend of Bach and Bush Essences, you can make up these remedies for menopause states:

Self-doubt	cerato, red grevillia, kapok bush, wild oat, and five corners
Hot flushes	cherry plum, impatiens, mimulus, walnut, billy goat plum, and mulla mulla
Anxiety	aspen, mimulus, larch, rock rose, crowea, and illawarra flame tree

Anger	cherry plum, holly, vine, rock water, and mountain devil
Irritability	beech, vervain, black-eyed Susan, and yellow cowslip orchid
Depression	cherry plum, gentian, gorse, mustard, white chestnut, wild rose, tall yellow top, and waratah
Self-conscious	crab apple, larch, wisteria, tall mulla mulla, and dog rose

WISE WOMAN WAYS

When using flower essences, it's important to use them in an integrated way. Don't just take them mindlessly. When I take a remedy, I consider why I'm taking it and what I can do to support myself in other ways. For example, if I'm taking a mixture for anger, I ask myself what or who is my anger directed at. What can I do to help externalize this feeling? What is it about? I might choose to journal my thoughts and feelings or talk them through with someone, taking the remedies as I consciously work through my issue.

How to Mix and Use Remedies

There are a variety of ways in which you can use the remedies:

Internal

Flower essences can be taken orally for acute cases by putting two or three drops of the stock bottle essence under the tongue. They can be taken longer-term by taking six drops from a dropper bottle that contains stock essence plus water.

To make up a remedy:

1. Fill a 20ml glass dropper bottle with tap or filtered water to a finger width beneath the neck of the bottle.
2. Choose your remedy (you can use a mixture of Australian Bush Essences and Bach Flower Remedies for up to six remedies). Drop two drops from the stock bottle into the dropper bottle.
3. If you are a Reiki practitioner, you might like to perform Reiki on the bottle.
4. Take four drops under the tongue, four times daily. Alternatively you can put the remedies in tea, coffee, fizzy drinks, and so on. If you are taking a made-up remedy, you might have four drops, four times daily for a period of one month or lunar cycle. Note: Putting the drops into a hot drink has the advantage of evaporating the alcohol. This is sometimes recommended for people who dislike the alcohol content or who are too sensitive to alcohol to take remedies containing it, such as those with adrenal issues.

Because of the dynamic nature of awakening and going to sleep at night, the most important times to take the remedy is immediately upon waking and before going to sleep. The other two times may be before lunch and around 6pm.

- INHALING: Put two drops of your chosen essence in the palm of your hands, rub them together and inhale from them.
- MEDITATION: One of the most powerful ways to use the essences is to take a few drops just before meditating.
- IN FOOD: When you make nourishing food for yourself, add your remedy to the food, either straight from the stock bottle or from your dropper bottle mixture.

WISE WOMAN WAYS

I find that taking the remedies is a multilayered opportunity for personal growth. When I feel distressed, I want the feelings to go away. I don't like feeling uncomfortable. I want to feel good. However, it isn't helpful to use the remedies as a "band-aid." Yes, the feelings may ease, but they may return again. Let's use anxiety as an example. Very often anxiety is the "acceptable face" we show the world. Anxiety, however, often covers up a range of other emotions that maybe aren't quite as "acceptable." Only the other day, I experienced feelings of being overwhelmed and anxious due to external pressures. I took myself off, did some relaxation exercises, a few stretches, and screamed into a cushion for good measure. There was the anger my anxiety had been holding down. So I took a remedy for the anger and helped myself through the blip.

External

- COMPRESS: This can be useful especially where there is a sore place or a chronic condition such as joint pain. Also, if it feels like there is a place in the body where, for instance, anger, grief, fear, or past trauma is being held, a compress may be a great comfort.

  To prepare a flower essence compress, fill a bowl with warm or cold water. Add four drops of each chosen flower essence (and four drops of appropriate essential oil if you like) to the water. Soak the flannel or cotton wool in the water, wring out and lay it on the affected area and repeat until relief is felt.

- BATHING: Run a bath. The water needs to be at body temperature or a little warmer. Add four drops of your chosen essence. Essential oils can also be added after the water is run. Get into the bath and relax for 20 minutes. Rest afterwards. If you don't want to have a bath, bathing the feet and/or hands is also an effective way to take essences in through the skin.

- BODY SPRAY: Adding essential oils to a body spray brings not only added healing benefits but also a wonderful uplifting smell. Lighter oils such as lavender, geranium, or lemongrass work best. To prepare a flower essence spray, fill a 50-125ml glass spray bottle with spring water. Add five drops of essential oil. Add three drops of each chosen flower essence. Shake the bottle to activate the essences, and spray twice daily, or as required.
- CHAKRA POINTS: With minimal knowledge of the chakra system, the seven wheel-shaped energy centers in the body, you can apply flower essences to a chakra area either directly from the stock bottle or take internally:

Chakra	Recommended Australian and Bach Flower Remedies
1. Root (base) chakra	Waratah, red lily (disconnection), sundew (indecisive), grey spider (panic), macrocarpa (exhaustion), rock rose (extreme panic and fears), clematis (daydreamer, ungrounded), hornbeam (mental exhaustion), aspen (vague fears of the unknown)
2. Sacral (spleen) chakra	Turkey bush (creativity), billy goat plum (releases shame), spinifex (cleansing, victim archetype), she oak (hormonal imbalance)

3. Solar plexus chakra	Old man banksia (counteracts weariness), macrocarpa (energy), crowea (releases worry), wild potato bush (releases feeling physically en-cumbered, weighted down), banksia robur (lethary), cerato (strength to trust one's own judgment, larch (lack of self-confidence), schleran-thus (indecisiveness)
4. Heart chakra	Bush fuchsia (speaking your true essence), crowea (worry), turkey bush (creativity), red grevillia (becoming unstuck), flannel flower (intimacy), illawara flame tree (fear of rejection), sturt desert pea (emotional pain), holly (blocked love), gorse (despair)
5. Throat chakra	Turkey bush (creative blocks)
6. Third-eye (brow) chakra	Bush iris (clears blocks relating to grounding and trust), bush fuscia (intuition), isopogon (memory)
7. Crown chakra	Red lily (disconnection), sundew (indecision), wild oat (reconnect-ing)

- CREAM/LOTION: If what you need is just for now, put some cream in your hand, add the required stock essences drops and mix before applying. To prepare a flower essence cream, fill a glass jar with 50g cream. You can use your favorite moisturizer as a base, but avoid any strongly scented creams. Add four drops of each chosen essence (up to four essences).

Mix cream and essence drops with a wooden stick or stiff drinking straw. A few drops of an essential oil can be added to the cream to enhance its healing properties. Apply to the area twice daily, or as required.

- HEALING: Put the remedy on your hands before doing energy work such as Reiki, Wiccan, or shamanic practices on yourself.
- MASSAGE: Mixing essences in massage oil can greatly enhance your mood. Put four drops of essential oil, four drops of relevant flower essence, and 50ml of jojoba oil into a glass bottle. Mix and use immediately. Recommended oils: lavender for anxiety, geranium for hot flushes, or ginger for fatigue.
- TO ENHANCE BODYWORK: Flower essences are powerful tools when used in conjunction with acupuncture, energy work, massage, craniosacral therapy, or chiropractic treatments. Taking a few drops of flower essences before, during, and/or after a treatment helps the body "hold" positive adjustments by assisting the nervous system with repatterning as well as releasing the emotional/mental blocks.
- SUBTLE ENERGY MASSAGE: Place a few drops of your chosen flower essence on your hands and give yourself a subtle energy massage.
  1. Keep your hands about two inches away from your body. Move your right hand from the heart area down the inside of your left arm and up the outside. Swap sides and do the same for the other arm.
  2. Move your hands over the heart area, up over the head to the neck, and round to under the chin. Move down to under the breast area, round to the back (kidney area), and down over the buttocks and the back of the legs, imagining the movement going under the feet.

3. Return your hands to the heart area and move both hands down over the torso and down the front of both legs, imagining the movement going under the feet.

- ROOMS: You could put a flower essence mixture in a bowl of water on the mantelpiece or table, or add your chosen oils to your burner and drop in four drops of flower essence. Another idea is to make up a spray as in the instructions for creating a body spray above and use on bedding or in a room.

What Happens Next?

While flower essences can contribute to improving our mindset, we can also develop the habit of relaxation and meditation as a useful mind-body skill. It can also enhance chakra healing, ritual, and quartz crystal healing. Curious? Turn the page, gentle reader.

CHAPTER 6

Relaxation and Meditation

You could record any of the following relaxations or meditations to reuse or ask someone to talk you through them.

Change and Stress

Menopause reflects a change in mind, body, and spirit. Siegelman (Siegelman,1983) [19] speculates that change is upsetting because we are leaving a part of ourselves behind. Any change involves a loss of the known. Siegelman also believes that there is an opposite force to the resistance to change. It is natural to seek change, to master new challenges, explore the unknown, and to test ourselves. From this we can gain access to new growth. The menopause years offers fantastic opportunities for change; however, when we look at the mind-body link, we can see how vulnerable we may be in this process of change.

Stress and Health

Stress describes our response to an event. The same event can happen to two people, and one may respond with a high level of stress symptoms while the other deals with the situation without any stress symptoms. Our perception of the event and our coping strategies determine how "stressed" we become. We might choose to believe that a "reasonable" amount of stress adds the edge of anticipation to life while too much or chronic stress can erode our psychological and physical resistance. We don't want to eliminate stress but to learn how to manage it.

Some of these signs of stress can also be symptomatic of menopause:

- PHYSICAL: erratic heart rate, increased sweating, headache, muscular pain, diarrhea/constipation, sickness, insomnia, fatigue, shallow breathing, recurrent infections, stomach ulcers, high blood pressure.
- EMOTIONAL: irritability, depression, reduced self-esteem, and anxiety.
- COGNITIVE: forgetfulness, lack of concentration, diminished sense of life meaning, and negative self-talk.
- BEHAVIOURAL: carelessness, increased eating/smoking/alcohol/drug use, withdrawal, listlessness, nervous laughter, loss of appetite, accident proneness, nail biting, and aggressive behaviour.

Menopause can contribute to chronic stress. The thought of change, and therefore potential threat, sends the message to our systems that our survival mechanisms of fight or flight need to be activated. The sympathetic nervous system responds to threatening events by diverting energy from internal organs to the muscles, heart rate increases, and the body is made ready for physical action. Energy cannot be diverted in both directions simultaneously, so when danger has been identified and the body makes a fight-or-flight response, the body suppresses the immune response temporarily in order to maximize the energy available to deal with the threat.

We know that the mind has a powerful impact on the body. Individuals who are chronically pessimistic, angry, or anxious tend to be more susceptible to stress and illness. Similarly, almost every medical condition affects people psychologically as well as physically (Hales, 2003).[20] Menopause isn't a medical condition; however, the changes in hormone levels associated with menopause can place stress on both body and mind.

All of the following conditions have been shown to have a stress component: asthma, chronic fatigue syndrome, tension headaches, depression, skin disorders, high blood pressure, fibromyalgia, insomnia, irritable bowel syndrome (IBS), menstrual difficulties, multiple sclerosis (MS), and ulcerative colitis. Psychological factors influence immune function, according to research into the importance of personal relationships. Researchers (Kiecolt-Glaser et al, 2002) [21] have detailed a range of conditions that suggest a psychological–immune-system link, including aging, cardiovascular disease, osteoporosis, arthritis, type 2 diabetes, and certain cancers.

The effect of a compromised immune system is even linked with breast cancer development. In research on women with metastatic breast cancer, psychiatrist David Spiegel found that stress hormones played a role in the progression of breast cancer (Spiegel, 2010).[22] The average survival time of women with normal cortisol patterns was significantly longer than that of women whose cortisol levels remained high throughout the day (an indicator of stress).

Relaxation and meditation are two self-help methods we can use to help ease our passage through the menopause years.

WISE WOMAN WAYS

Learning to recognize and manage excess stress is an incredibly useful life skill. A certain amount of stress keeps us going, but too much and we can be in deep doo-doo. I can tell when I'm approaching my stress threshold. My body becomes clenched including teeth and hair follicles! My breathing becomes shallow. I'm irritable above and beyond the call of duty. And I might get a cold or not sleep well.

How do YOU recognize when you're overstretched? More importantly: What do you do about it?

Relaxation Through Better Breathing

When stressed, breathing becomes shallow. There are normally two ways of breathing, chest or abdominal. Chest breathing is shallow, irregular, and fast, and the body does not receive the correct amount of oxygen. A tipoff to this is that a person will continually sigh, as a means of getting extra oxygen into the system, which provides short-term relief. This type of pattern often causes a person to hold their breath, hyperventilate, and experience shortness of breath. On top of this, the stress response will be activated hence more anxiety, and more shallow breathing. This type of breathing is also associated with mouth breathing, which the body immediately associates with stress. Breathing through the nose automatically soothes the system and leads to fuller belly breathing.

The other main way for breathing is abdominal, or belly, breathing. Belly breathing is the way we are supposed to breathe and a sign of health. Just watch a newborn baby breathing and you will see; it is adults who forget how to do this. On inhaling through the nose, the lungs open fully to allow as much oxygen to enter the system. The diaphragm contracts and expands to allow the lungs to expand, which naturally causes the belly to push out. This means the body has the right levels of oxygen to provide energy.

Abdominal breathing

Abdominal breathing can be very soothing because it slows you down. It is also efficient, bringing a good supply of oxygen to your brain. Check your breathing pattern by putting one hand on your chest and one hand on your stomach. If your lower hand moves and your top hand does not, you are doing abdominal breathing. But if your top hand moves and your bottom one does not, you are doing chest breathing.

Let's do some abdominal breathing. You're going to inhale through your nose and exhale out of your mouth. Your exhalation needs to be longer than your inhalation. To slow your exhalation down, let your breath gently out, just enough to flicker a candle (purse your lips).

- Lay down flat and place your hands fingertip to fingertip, with your middle fingers meeting at your belly button.
- As you inhale through your nose, push your belly up and feel your fingertips expand. Rest a beat, before exhaling slowly through your mouth. Rest a beat before inhaling again and feel your belly rise. Repeat this cycle five times.
- Now place your hands under the breast area of each side of your body, which is the rib area.
- As you inhale through your nose, expand your ribs and feel your hands push out. Rest a beat, before exhaling slowly through your mouth. Rest a beat before inhaling again and feel your ribs expand. Repeat this cycle five times.
- Now you are going to do a complete breathing cycle, inhaling deeply from the belly and ribcage and exhaling completely.
- As you inhale through your nose for a count of five, push your belly up and expand your ribs. Rest a beat, before exhaling slowly through your mouth for a count of six. Rest a beat before inhaling again and feel your belly rise and your ribs expand. Repeat this cycle five times.

The more you practice abdominal breathing, the easier it will become. Eventually, you will be able to do it anywhere—sitting, standing, or lying down.

Body Scan

Sit or lay down in a comfortable place where you won't be disturbed and close your eyes. Take in a slow, deep breath through your nose and exhale completely. And again. Allow your body to become comfortable as you breathe deeply and easily.

Place your awareness in your forehead and scalp. Allow any tension in the forehead and scalp to drain over the back of the head and out of the base of your neck into infinity. You're breathing easily and deeply. Releasing and relaxing. Your eyes are gently closed. Ease away the frown. Wiggle your jaw from side to side to loosen the tension. Your tongue should be behind your lower teeth. You're breathing easily and deeply.

- Focus your awareness on your right shoulder and arm. Allow any tension in the right shoulder and arm to drain down the arm. Down, down, down the arm, out the fingers, and into infinity.
- Focus your awareness on your left shoulder and arm. Allow any tension in the left shoulder and arm to drain down the arm. Down, down, down the arm, out the fingers, and into infinity. You're breathing easily and deeply. Releasing and relaxing.
- Focus on the chest area. Feel the chest area opening and expanding. You're breathing easily and deeply.
- Focus on the stomach. Allow the stomach to relax. Releasing and relaxing.
- Focus your awareness on the back area. Upper back, middle back, and lower back. Allow any tension in the back area to slide down the spine. Down, down, down the spine, out the base of the spine, into infinity. You're breathing easily and deeply. Releasing and relaxing.
- Focus your attention on your right hip and leg. Allow any tension in the right hip and leg to drain down the leg. Down, down, down the leg, out the toes, into infinity.
- Focus your attention on your left hip and leg. Allow any

tension in the left hip and leg to drain down the leg. Down, down, down the leg, out the toes, into infinity. Releasing and relaxing.

• You feel completely relaxed from head to toe—more relaxed than you have been in a long while.

> **WISE WOMAN WAYS**
>
> Journaling your way through menopause can be incredibly helpful. I've used journaling throughout my adult life—when I had breast cancer, through relationship difficulties, family issues, and work crisis. All you need is paper and pen. Your command of English doesn't matter—only your intent to externalize your thoughts and feelings. No one else need read your words or gaze on your doodling. Journaling has helped me work through problems and externalize difficult personal thoughts I wouldn't dream of telling anyone.

Mindfulness Meditation

Mindfulness is being aware of the present moment. We tend to trap ourselves in between future fear and past guilt. Maybe we go into the past or future to escape an uncomfortable present, such as personal difficulties or illness. We practice mindfulness meditation to live life more meaningfully in the present moment.

The meditation

Find yourself a comfortable position and close your eyes. Bring your attention to the present moment and focus on your breath, breathing normally and naturally. You can place your awareness either at the tip of your nose or upon your abdomen. If you're focusing on the tip of the nose, feel the touch of cool air up your nostrils and down your throat as you inhale and the warmth of air as you exhale. If you're focusing on the abdomen, feel the belly push upwards on inhaling and contract on exhaling.

Be aware of each inhalation and each exhalation. Watch the breath going in and out without judgment. Be in the present, and notice the breath. Breathing in. Breathing out. Watch each breath appear and disappear. Merely breathing.

Let go of your awareness of the breath and bring your attention to your body. Feel and observe without judgment. Acknowledge the multitude of sensations moment to moment. If there are areas in the body where there is discomfort, allow it to ease if possible. If the discomfort remains, then let it be there and observe the sensations. Observe your body without judgment. Sensations come, sensations go. Watch them appear, stay, or disappear. Merely sensations.

Let go of your awareness of sensations and bring your attention to your mind. To your thoughts and emotions. Observe the mind without judgment. Acknowledge the multitude of mental shapes moment to moment. As if you were standing by the sea, watching the tide come in and go out, watch the mind in the same way. Thoughts come, thoughts go. Watch them appear, stay, or disappear. Merely thoughts.

Let go of your awareness of the mind and bring your attention to your hearing. Observe the sounds without judgment. Acknowledge the multitude of varying sounds internally or externally. Moment to moment, sounds come and sounds go. Watch them appear and disappear. Merely sounds.

Returning to the breath and feeling the whole body as you breathe in and out. Feel the whole of your body expand with an inhalation and contract on an exhalation. Becoming more mindful of your body. Of the room that you are in. When you are ready open your eyes, feeling however you choose to feel.

WISE WOMAN WAYS

Incredibly easy ways to chill:

- Going for a walk with no aim in mind, nothing to do and no money on you to buy anything (apart from maybe a cup of tea!)

- Tuck yourself up in a quiet and comfortable place and go to sleep in the middle of the day.

- Indulge in a spell of comfort food, such as mashed potato with cheese, tomato soup, hot chocolate... well, you know the kind of thing.

- Buy something you have always wanted, can afford, and is a total waste of time and money—but it makes you incredibly happy.

- When I've had enough, I like to crash out with a steaming, roller coaster of a novel, a packet of crunchy potato crisps, and a really green apple. Or how about chocolate raisons? There again, maybe a glass of something bubbly... Mind you, there's nothing like having your feet massaged and stroked. Did I tell you I really enjoy having my head scratched for that chill-out sensation?

Wise Woman Meditation

Find somewhere comfortable and quiet to sit or lay, preferably in nature. Close your eyes and focus on your body. Take a deep breath through your nose, hold for a beat, before exhaling through your mouth. Make your exhalation longer than your inhalation. Take another couple of deep breaths. Take your time to scan your body and release any tension. All the while, breathing deeply and easily.

Allow your body to relax. If you notice any areas of discomfort or tension that are difficult to let go of, accept them as best you can and focus your mind on your breath. Deeply inhaling, resting for a beat, then exhaling completely. Rest a beat before inhaling once more. You're breathing deeply and easily, focusing your mind on your breathing.

Imagine that you're lying beneath an ancient oak tree, on a warm summer night. The grass is soft beneath you, there is a cool breeze across your forehead, and you can hear the leaves above rustle quietly. As you look up through the branches of the oak tree, you can see the night sky and stars. High above, the full moon reaches down between the branches, shining on you and reaching deep into your heart. With each breath, you draw in more and more of the moonlight, as it floods your body and mind. It soaks through you, spilling into the earth.

The moonlight permeates every cell and every organ of your body, relaxing and renewing you with each breath you take. Your body is completely relaxed, warm, and heavy. Feel yourself sinking into the earth. Deeper into the earth. You're sinking deep into the earth. Relaxing even more with each breath you take. Imagine that you are deep within the earth. The nurturing, nourishing energy of the earth surrounds you. Imagine that you are in a place that is very familiar to you. In your mind's eye, open to the woodland scene around you. It is early morning, and the light is just beginning to warm the air, as you rise and walk along the path, feeling secure and peaceful. As the path winds through the trees, you come to a small stream and pause for a moment to notice it before stepping over to the other side. Once on the other side, the path continues, leading you to a home that you know well—a place where you have been many times before. It is the home of your Wise Woman.

As you are about to knock, the door swings open and your Wise Woman greets you with a loving hug. Her home feels warm and loving. She leads you to the kitchen, where she has cooked for you. You sit with her and, while sharing food, speak with her about this time in your life when your mind, body, and spirit are changing to become the Wise Woman yourself.

Times passes, and it is early evening. Your Wise Woman leads you from the kitchen to the back door. You open the door and walking through, you step out into a woodland clearing. In the centre of the clearing a small altar is set up, and you go and sit in front of it, adding anything to it that you may have brought with you.

Your Wise Woman sits across from you and asks you what you need to know about this sacred time in your life. You are able to ask her any questions, and in this place, you are able to hear the true answers. In turn, your Wise Woman asks you questions, which you are able to answer with your truth. When all the questions have been answered, she reaches down onto the altar and picks up an object to give to you—one that will remind you of the truth about your inner Wise Woman. You take it and put it in your pocket. You can stay as long as you like, resting in this place.

When you are ready, your Wise Woman leads you through the back door and out to the front of the house. She gives you a hug goodbye, and while in her embrace, whispers one word or phrase that will help you to remember your intentions for this time in your life and what you need to do to make them manifest as you travel through the Change. You thank her and head back to the path, drinking in the feeling of peace and home. You step across the stream again, heading back towards the path that brought you here.

As you walk along the path, you feel calm, positive, and relaxed. You are one with the earth and all of nature around you. You're breathing easily and deeply as you sink into the earth once more and begin the transformation to return to lying back down on the grass where you began, under the beautiful oak gazing up at the full moon in the night sky. Lay there for a while, reorientating yourself. Become aware of your body, your fingers and toes. Take in a deep breath and release. When you are ready, open your eyes and come back to the now, bringing your inner Wise Woman with you.

WISE WOMAN WAYS

Incredibly easy meditations include:

- Lay in the grass watching the clouds through sleepy eyes.
- Lay on the beach with closed eyes, listening to the surf and the muted sounds of people around you.
- Lay under a tree.
- Paddle along the seashore's edge—as far as you can, as long as you like.
- Take a long walk by a long river.

What Happens Next?

Now that you have a relaxed mind and body, you may feel so chilled, that you can't even turn the next page. However, if you don't turn the page, you might miss out on how chakra healing can further enrich your menopause years.

Useful Resources

- *www.wisdomofthecrone.com* (a deck of 54 wisdom cards, each bearing a unique image of women between the ages of 50 and 100, useful for meditation and reflection)

CHAPTER 7

Chakra Healing

Think of yourself as an eclectic energy field of mind, body, and spirit—mind, with its intellect and emotions; the physical body; and the elusive spirit. Spiritual energy is less tangible, yet it permeates and underpins all the other energy fields. In addition to healing the mind and body during the menopause years, we need to look at nourishing the energetic body that is part of our spiritual nature.

To grasp spiritual energy, we need to have some concept of the divine or the sacred. These two words could be defined as the infinite, the everlasting, God, Goddess, or universal energy. We may reflect that our human connection to the sacred is through our sense of spirituality, like an umbilical cord.

Our awareness of our spirituality, our connection to the divine, develops throughout our lifetime (or several). Metaphorically, you might consider your spirituality as a flame deep within you that as you become more conscious, burns brighter.

WISE WOMAN WAYS

When I teach students about energetic anatomy, I explain it this way. Imagine you are a ball of light. This is your eternal flame, your link with the sacred, your spiritual self. In order for its brightness and connectedness to grow, you need to become increasingly aware of the defenses it has around it that dim its glow—defenses such as ego, anger, fear, and so on.

As you become more aware of yourself and work to let go of the mindsets that hold you back, more of these defenses will begin to fall away, allowing the ball of light to burn brighter still, increasing your connectedness to the sacred.

Imagine covering this ball of light in something like a loose-weave cloth. You can see the cloth, but because the weave is so loose, you can also see the glow of the ball through the cloth. This cloth represents your energetic anatomy, your auric field and chakra system. Energetic anatomy isn't a physical thing; it's a subtle energy manifestation and is as important as your physical anatomy. The energy field is like a multi-gateway system, through which you give and receive mental, emotional, physical, and spiritual energy. The more your ball glows and grows, the more the weave of your energy field expands. The development of your energetic anatomy and your ball of light become increasingly one and the same.

The chakra system is part of your energy anatomy system and consists of several major chakras and many minor chakras. The word *chakra* is a Sanskrit word, meaning "vortex" or "wheel." These chakras aren't on the physical body but on the etheric body (part of your auric energy field). A major chakra resembles a spinning wheel. When balanced, it spins appropriately. If the chakra is blocked, the spin may be slower or static. When overstimulated, the chakra may be spinning too fast.

Each chakra has a relationship to our physical body as well as to psychological mindsets. Our chakra system evolves as we grow older. This chapter will help you engage with chakra healing, as you travel through the menopause years.

The Chakra System

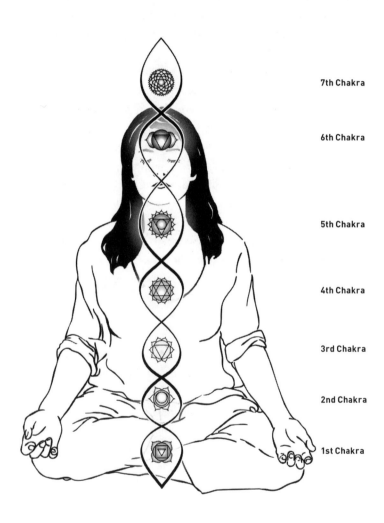

7th Chakra

6th Chakra

5th Chakra

4th Chakra

3rd Chakra

2nd Chakra

1st Chakra

Grounding Yourself

Before starting to perform any type of chakra healing, it is important to ground yourself. Grounding allows you to remain firmly connected to the earth by perceiving yourself anchored by roots that extend down to the core of the earth via your root/base chakra, for example. It prevents you from feeling "floaty" or "spaced out."

A grounding exercise

Sit or stand with eyes closed and observe your breathing for a few minutes. Visualize yourself as a tree, with roots growing down into the earth through the soles of your feet. The energy of your being roots deep into the earth and any excess energy is grounded within your strong roots. When you feel you are sufficiently anchored or earthed, bring yourself back into the room.

Other grounding techniques include: tai chi breathing, yogic breathing, physical exercise, eating something, being in nature, putting your hands into sand, soil, or running water.

Protecting Yourself

Whenever we are consciously working with our chakras, we open ourselves up to receiving the universal healing energy and are more sensitive to the energies around us. To protect against unwanted negative or draining energies, there are a number of techniques you can use.

A protection exercise

Wrap a protective cloak of light and vitality around yourself, covering head to toe. Visualize it as any colour that offers strength, comfort, and reassurance. Request that universal energy, God, or Goddess protect you from all negative energy.

Cleansing Yourself

Our chakras need cleansing regularly to get rid of unwanted energies absorbed from people, places, or situations. If you are feeling tired, drained, or emotionally unstable, you may be absorbing and carrying external energies. Daily cleansing will help to clear these energies and improve the circulation of your own energies.

It is also important to make sure that you have carried out a cleansing exercise before you self-heal. The clearer your chakras and aura are, the more healing energy you will be able to create, attract, and absorb.

A cleansing exercise

First ground and protect yourself. Smudge sticks are a traditional way of cleansing, using a bound stick of sage and sweetgrass. Light the smudge stick and wave it around your body to cleanse your physical body, your aura, and chakras. Now start to get a sense of your aura. Feel how far it extends out into the space around you. See and sense its layers with your inner vision. Ask the divine for the love and light within your aura to be expanded to the appropriate level for you at this time. Ask that any negative energies be removed instantly and immediately, absorbed back into the divine and dissolved into light. Ask the divine to cleanse, heal, and protect you. Once this cleansing exercise is complete, bring your focus back to your breathing and your physical body.

> **WISE WOMAN WAYS**
>
> All this grounding, protecting, and cleansing can sound a tad woolly; however, an awareness of your subtle energy and a willingness to engage with it in a practical way will help you feel calmer and more positive. I can't guarantee that, of course! Try it and see for yourself.

Working With the Chakras
During the Menopause Years

CHAKRA	1
Yin and Yang poles	Yin (receptive and feminine)
Location	Base of spine between anus and genitals, connected to coccyx and opening downwards
Sensory function	Smell
Associated body parts	Skeletal system, adrenal glands, kidneys, anus, prostate, bladder, and genitals
Physical dysfunction	Osteoporosis and adrenal fatigue
Life issues	Survival, physical needs, standing up for oneself, physical health and fitness, grounding, stability, security, group power, and identity
Emotional dysfunction	Mental lethargy, "spaciness," victim mentality, unfocused mind, and distrust
Behaviourial dysfunction	Difficulty achieving goals, overactive, passivity, not looking after one's body
Colour	Red/black
Element	Earth
Bush Essence Flowers	Waratah, red lily (disconnection), sundew (indecisive), fringe violet (aura damage), grey spider (panic), macrocarpa (exhaustion), and bush iris (clearing blocks of physical excess and materialism)

Bach Flower Remedies	Rock rose (extreme panic and fears), clematis (daydreamer, too much time in the spirit realm, ungrounded), hornbeam (mental exhaustion), aspen (vague fears of the unknown)
Aromatherapy oils	Sandalwood, cedarwood, patchouli, myrrh, musk, lavender
Quartz crystals	Red tiger's eye, garnet, red jasper, ruby, obsidian, hematite, agate, bloodstone, garnet, red coral, ruby, hematite, onyx, rose quartz, smoky quartz
Yoga positions	Bridge, half and full locust, spinal roll, balancing, child pose

Reflections

- What are your physical needs at this point in time?
- What do you do for physical fitness?
- How do you recognize when you need grounding? What do you do in order to ground yourself?
- What gives you stability and security?
- Have you focused on abundance or lack today?
- How effective are you at setting and achieving goals? Are you able to put your thoughts into action?

I recognize when this chakra is out because I can get lower back pain and constipation, while psychologically I know that I'm not trusting myself or another person about something. If you excuse the pun, this chakra for me can be a pain the bum!

CHAKRA	2
Yin and Yang poles	Yang (positive and masculine)
Location	Lower abdomen, between naval and genitals, opens forward
Sensory function	Taste
Associated body parts	Circulatory system, uterus, ovaries, and testes glands
Physical dysfunction	Impotence, frigidity, bladder and prostate trouble, lower back pain, and erratic libido
Life issues	Emotional balance, sexuality, uncovering motivations, influencing choices based on conditioning, allowing pleasure, creative expression, partnerships, and playfulness
Emotional dysfunction	Instability, sadness, feelings of isolation, and martyr mentality
Behaviourial dysfunction	Excessive libido, sexual withdrawal
Colour	Orange
Element	Water
Yoga positions	Cobra, pelvic rock, goddess pose, leg lifts, pelvic side rolls, downward facing dog, open legs, and hip circles
Aromatherapy oils	Melissa, orange, mandarin, neroli, sandalwood, ylang ylang, jasmine, and rose
Australian Bush Essences	Turkey bush (creativity), billy goat plum (releases shame), spinifex (cleansing, victim artchtype), she oak (hormonal imbalance), and

	flannel flower (lack of sensitivity, especially in males, and sexual abuse)
Bach Flower Remedies	Agrimony, centaury, pine, larch, and gorse
Quartz crystals	Coral, carnelian, citrine, and golden topaz

Reflections

- What influences do you still carry from your past that influence current life choices?
- How do you know when you are emotionally unbalanced or in balance?
- How do you express creativity?
- Are your sexual relationships mutual and respectful? How do you relate to your sexuality?
- To what extent to you live in the present moment?

Ah, the chakra of creative self-expression. At the time of writing this book, when my uterus has a fluid life of its own—my creative side is struggling to be birthed on a more profound level. I've never birthed a physical baby, but by jingo, birthing the baby of creativity surely comes a close second!

CHAKRA	3
Yin and Yang poles	Yin (receptive and feminine)
Location	Between naval and base of sternum, opens forward
Sensory function	Sight
Associated body parts	Digestive system, gallbladder, spleen, pancreas, liver, limbic system, and adrenal glands

Physical dysfunction	Stomach ulcers, fatigue, weight around stomach, allergies, and diabetes
Life issues	Personal power, will, self-esteem/self-confidence, the courage to take risks, to be, purpose, effectiveness, endurance, self-respect, uniqueness, and individuality
Emotional dysfunction	Oversensitive to criticism, low self-esteem
Behavioural dysfunction	Aggressive, controlling, addictions
Colour	Yellow
Element	Fire
Aromatherapy oils	Rosemary, lemon, grapefruit, bergamot, ginger, rose, ylang ylang, and cinnamon
Yoga positions	Bow, pike pose, belly push, boat pose, front stretch, warrior
Australian Bush Essences	Dynamis essence (combination of essences for energy), old man banksia (counteracts weariness), macrocarpa (energy), crowea (releases worry), wild potato bush (releases feeling physically encumbered, weighted down), banksia robur (lethargy), bottlebrush (bonding between mother and child, letting go), peach flowered tea tree, waratah, five corners
Bach Flower Remedies	Cerato (strength to trust one's own judgment), larch (lack of self-

	confidence), schleranthus (indecisiveness), chicory, larch, pine, crab apple, and walnut
Quartz crystals	Citrine, amber, tiger's eye, yellow topaz

Reflections

- How would you rate your self-esteem?
- What was the last risk you took? How do you feel about it now?
- Do you lack confidence? Are you overly concerned with what other people think?
- How do you rate your decision-making skills?
- Do you take on too much responsibility?
- How do you relate to your personal power? Do you need to become more assertive?

> **WISE WOMAN WAYS**
>
> Continue to develop a conscious awareness of your energetic anatomy. Sometimes I can be doing something inane and I become aware that my hand chakras are generating enormous heat. Waste not, want not—I channel this active healing energy to those in need.

CHAKRA	4
Yin and Yang poles	Yang (positive and masculine)
Location	Centre of chest (breastbone), opens forward
Sensory function	Feeling
Associated body parts	Heart, chest, lungs, circulation, and thymus gland

Physical dysfunction	Shallow breathing, high blood pressure, heart disease, and cancer
Life issues	Beliefs about love and relationships, forgiveness and compassion for oneself and others, balance, compassion and self-acceptance, and unconditional acceptance of others
Emotional dysfunction	Co-dependency, melancholia, fears concerning loneliness, commitment, and/or betrayal
Behaviourial dysfunction	Passivity, withdrawal
Colour	Green/pink
Element	Air
Yoga positions	Cobra, the fish, cow-face, breathing techniques
Quartz crystals	Aventurine, emerald, jade, malachite, peridot, rose quartz, watermelon tourmaline, green calcite, azurite, and moonstone
Australian Bush Essences	Bush fuchsia (speaking your true essence), crowea (worry), turkey bush (creativity), red grevillia (becoming unstuck), flannel flower (intimacy), illawara flame tree (fear of rejection), sturt desert pea (emotional pain), bluebell, rough bluebell, waratah
Bach Flower Remedies	Holly (blocked love), gorse (despair), chicory
Aromatherapy oils	Eucalyptus, pine, tea tree, cedarwood, rose, jasmine, rose, bergamot, and melissa

Reflections

- Do you accept yourself for who you are or do you lack self-love?
- Are you compassionate, or do you judge others?
- Do you respond to others through your mind and intellect rather than your heart?
- Consider a relationship where you may have been co-dependent. What was it like for you?
- Do you have a fear of being rejected or abandoned?
- How do you show commitment in relationships? What conditions do you tend to put onto a relationship?

This heart chakra is, for me, maybe the most poignant of all. To experience self-love and self-respect is most challenging. Yet how can we truly love another or accept love from another, if we don't have this love and respect for the self?

CHAKRA	5
Yin and Yang poles	Yin (receptive and feminine)
Location	Centrally at base of neck, opens forward
Sensory function	Hearing
Associated body parts	Throat, ears, nose teeth, mouth, neck, thyroid, and parathyroid glands
Physical dysfunction	Sore throats, neck ache, thyroid problems, hearing problems, tinnitus, and asthma
Life issues	Communication, self-expression, the power of choice, personal expression, harmony with others, self-knowledge, creativity

Emotional dysfunction	Perfectionism, inability to express emotions, and blocked creativity
Behaviourial dysfunction	Withdrawal, people pleasing
Colour	Light blue
Element	Sound
Bach Flower Remedies	Agrimony
Australian Bush Essences	Cognis essence (clarity and courage to speak truth, great for study and new information), paw paw (assimilating new information), turkey bush (creative blocks), old man banksia, flannel flower, bush fuchsia, mint bush
Quartz crystals	Sodalite, lapis lazuli, blue agate, aquamarine, turquoise, celestite, sapphire
Aromatherapy oils	Geranium, chamomile, myrrh, peppermint, mint, cypress, lavender or bergamot
Yoga positions	Neck rolls, shoulder stand, fish pose, the plough

Reflections

- Are you able to express yourself and your beliefs (voice your inner truth)?
- Are you able to free yourself of old family values, beliefs, and commitments, especially regarding their relationship to responsibility?
- What life roles or masks do you hide behind?
- How do you express your emotions?

Many years ago in my late twenties, I went through a particular growth phase when I was making connections with my "little Laurel" side and realizing how much of my inappropriate adult drives were happening because of unhealthy childhood conditioning. In one vision quest, I saw myself as a thin, naked little girl with a paper bag over her head. In the two weeks following this, I developed a cold and a horrendous cough, during which time (I hope this isn't too much information for you) phlegm caught in my throat by the bucketful necessitating an emergency visit by the doctor. My cough and cold came and went. More importantly, I learnt to express my feelings as an adult and to heal from past trauma.

CHAKRA	6
Yin and Yang poles	Yang (receptive and masculine
Location	Above and between eyebrows, opens forward
Sensory function	Sixth sense
Associated body parts	Eyes, base of skull, nose, ears, and pituitary gland
Physical dysfunction	Headaches, poor vision, neurological disturbances, glaucoma, and nightmares
Life issues	Intuition, wisdom, emotional intelligence, ability to "see" other than with the eyes
Emotional dysfunction	Seasonally depressed
Behaviourial dysfunction	Learning difficulties, hallucinations
Colour	Indigo
Element	Light
Australian Bush Essences	Bush iris (clears blocks relating to grounding and trust), bush fuchsia

	(intuition), isopogon (memory), green spider orchid, and boronia
Bach Flower Remedies	Walnut, crab apple, rock water, and vervain
Quartz crystals	Tourmaline, tanzanite, lapis lazuli, sapphire, amethyst, purple apatite, azurite, calcite, and fluorite
Aromatherapy oils	Patchouli, frankincense, myrrh, bergamot, hyacinth, violet, and rose geranium
Yoga positions	Palming, seated yoga mudra visualization and imagery.

Reflections

- How might you develop your intuitive abilities?
- How much silence is there in your life for the whispers of intuition to be heard?
- How do you balance your imagination and fantasy realm with reality?
- To what extent do you hide your intuition behind a rational mind?

CHAKRA	7
Yin and Yang poles	Yin and Yang
Location	Top/crown of head, opens upward
Sensory function	None
Associated body parts	Upper skull, cerebral cortex, skin, pineal gland
Physical dysfunction	Sensitivity to pollution, chronic exhaustion, epilepsy, and Alzheimer's disease

Life issues	Spirituality, selflessness, expanded consciousness
Emotional dysfunction	Depression, obsessional thinking, confusion
Behaviourial dysfunction	Obsessive-compulsive disorder (OCD)
Colour	Violet, white, and gold
Element	Thought, cosmic energy
Australian Bush Essences	Red lily (disconnection), sundew (indecision), angelsword, bush iris, and waratah
Bach Flower Remedies	Wild oat (reconnecting)
Aromatherapy oils	Lavender, frankincense, and rosewood
Yoga positions	Headstand, seated meditation
Quartz crystals	Amethyst, diamond, clear quartz, white jade, white tourmaline, snowy quartz, and herkimer.

Reflections

- When was the last time you did a selfless act?

What Happens Next?

Working with your subtle energy is a creative process that can be taken to even greater depths through sexual healing. Read on to discover how you can enrich your sexual journey through menopause.

CHAPTER 8

Sexual Journeys

What did you learn at the knee of your mother (or father) about sexuality? When I was in my teens and experienced climaxes in my dreams, I asked Mum what it was all about, and received my answer in her panic-stricken stare and pursed lips. Ah, back to my teen magazines then, to glean the only understanding available. I didn't talk about it with friends, as they (and I) were too embarrassed to discuss it… either that, or they were already engaged in sexual activities raunchy enough to make your hair curl.

Apart from some knee-trembling moments with different boys, I remained fairly unsullied until I met my husband when I was 19. I shall always remember his wonderful shock, as he was about to go where no man had gone before, when I announced I was still a virgin. If you excuse the way I put it: I am sure he would have framed and mounted me, such was his sweet delight. Thirty-two years later, we are still together.

The journey of sexuality is an evocative one. As young children, we learn overtly or covertly about our bodies and sex. As we grow up we have our myths and beliefs surrounding both the sexual relationship with ourselves and the sexual act with others. Our teen years may have been filled with erotic or ignorant fumblings (with self and others). Hormones rampant, maturity not always obvious, and understanding somewhat lacking, we move into adulthood still carrying our sexual myths and beliefs. These may include:

- Sex is mainly for procreation;
- Sex will bring the attention and affection we lacked in childhood;

- Sex is dirty;
- Sex is a physical release;
- Sex is a healthy and natural act.

As we grow older and become more life-experienced, our beliefs and emotions around sex affect how we engage with the act itself. As we travel through the menopause years, our sexual expression gives us the gift of mellowing from pure lust to sexual pleasure woven with love, spiritual insight, and Wise Woman wisdom.

WISE WOMAN WAYS

YONI is the Sanskrit word for the female genital area and is symbolic of the Universal Womb or the Great Mother Goddess (Gaia), from which creation emerges and dissolves back into.

LINGAM is the Sanskrit word for the male penis and is symbolic of the supreme life force. An erect penis evokes creative power poised for new life.

When you remain mindful of the greater symbolism of your sexual organs, it can heighten intimacy and unite mind, body and spirit and result in the expression of sacred sexuality.

Being in a Long-Term Relationship

In the years between my early 20s and late 30s, my husband and I would make love passionately and often. Lovingly unleashed, our sexuality was wonderfully creative. Over the 32 years we have been together, the sharp clarity of passion has changed to muted pastels of gentle lust, tempered with heart and soul. As we women move through menopause, we need to understand better how our sexual needs have changed and the way they need to be expressed now. Intense emotions are likely to give way to softer expression. As we move through the menopause years, our life experience, thoughts, and feelings begin to be outwardly reflected. The more we are in tune with ourselves, the clearer our inner balance shines through our physicality.

If you are in a long-term relationship, reflect on how the interaction between you has changed over the years and how this has influenced your sexual expression. If you are experiencing relationship difficulties, the sexual side of things may be challenging. If you feel angry or tense with your partner, then intimacy can be difficult to achieve.

Your partner is getting older as well. They may be experiencing physical or psychological issues that affect their lovemaking; this, in turn, impacts their relationship with you. As men become older their sex drive can naturally decrease, leading you to wonder if he still desires you and making you question your own attractiveness.

WISE WOMAN WAYS

The Five Phases of a Woman's Monthly Menstrual Cycle [23]

According to Mahasatvaa Ma Ananda Sarita, a woman's sexual cycle flows with the waxing and waning moon. This cycle is expressed in the following ways:

- From the end of menstruation through to the 10th day, a woman is physiologically and psychologically like a young girl (Maiden) wanting to flirt and be sexually playful.
- From days 10 to 18, she is a sexual and fertile young woman ready to conceive (Mother).
- From days 18 until four days before menstruation, she is in the middle-aged phase of reflection (Crone).

- Four days before menstruation until the beginning of menstruation, a woman experiences the "premenstrual flush," a time when life energies burst into a creative outpouring that reflects the past month's experiences.

Note: I believe that the way a woman psychologically experiences her menstrual cycle reflects larger social messages about permissible ways to express female emotions. It's all too easy to become bad-tempered or withdraw in an anxious state because it's "period time" and we feel we are allowed to conveniently dump difficult feelings into the category of "PMS"; in fact, how we handle our emotions the rest of the time is the real issue.

Talking sex

Talking sex with a partner needs openness, honesty, and tact. A male partner's ego tends to be more tied up with sex than a woman's is, and they may not always be as open as they could be when listening to their partner's thoughts and feeling around the sexual act and body image.

Sex isn't just about orgasm, yours or your partner's. There needs to be time to allow intimacy to build, so sharing your thoughts with your partner on how to bring quality rather than quantity to the art of lovemaking may be useful. Criticism is not the way forward! It's not about telling him he's not doing it right; you need to talk with him about how he could do it even better by… (I'll leave this space for you to get as creative as you like). Get the idea?

Men and women's take on sex

Men have a different take on sex than women. For most males, there is the mental and physical excitement, followed by physical release and satisfaction, all blended together with the motivation of possession. Women need preamble and intimacy. While a good quickie can be a turn-on, women also appreciate the tenderness of foreplay (wine, roses, food, and the G-spot!), as well as the psychological and spiritual connection. While physical contact for most men means sex, women enjoy cuddling, stroking, and touching—not only as a prelude to sex but often just as a loving expression in itself.

Life getting in the way of sex

Life worries can affect libido. If I'm ticked off with my husband, there is no way I can get down to brass tacks or let him into my most sacred of spaces. If I'm worried about something, my mind is elsewhere and couldn't possibly encompass looking sexy and hanging upside down from the chandelier.

Hormonal changes

Decreased libido may reflect hormonal changes, which may be rectified through the judicious use of herbs. Changing hormones may also give rise to vaginal dryness, which again could be improved through the use of herbs. Vaginal dryness may also be due to your state of mind about your body image, about your sexual needs, or about your relationship.

WISE WOMAN WAYS

Rising In Love [24]

As we travel the path of being in love through the menopause years, lovemaking can become habitual and not as nourishing as it could be. "Rising in Love," a concept described by Mahasatvaa Ma Ananda Sarita in her book *Divine Sexuality*, weaves together biology and mind in the service of your higher self.

Rising in Love blends exploration and higher wisdom into the sexual act, taking it beyond genital release. She suggests these tips:

- Show your appreciation for your lover through words, eye contact, touch, and actions.
- Make the nurturing of your relationship a priority.
- Create space for new styles of lovemaking, including tantra. Tantra emerged from two religions of ancient India: Shakti, whose roots can be traced to the Mother Goddess and fertility rites, and Shiva, the masculine equivilent. Both celebrate the sacred within the mundane—the spirit within the body. Enjoying tantric sexual practices with your partner can bring the divine (the Shakti and the Shiva) into the sexual.

Your changing needs

What you wanted from a sexual relationship when you were in your 20s won't be the same as in your 40s or 50s. I remember how I used to physically feel desire and passion when I was young as wonderfully sharp jabs in the womb and vagina area. Over recent years, those feeling have all but disappeared. This evaporation led me to believe the desire and passion weren't there. However, I've since learnt to recognize softer signs of passion and desire within me.

Body image

Body image can be an issue for the woman going through her menopause years. I look down over my one or two chins and crane my neck (only slightly) to see my furry slipper-encased feet. Why should I have to put up with cold feet? What else can I tell you about my body image? My left boob is a rebuild from when I had breast cancer 13 years ago. My right boob is lower than my left and is scarred from the reduction in order to match my other boob. Moving down over the curve of my belly (bloat, wheat intolerance, whatever), I see my legs as not too bad, albeit a tad knock-kneed. I won't bore you with any other details. Suffice to say that my body isn't ideal, and nor is yours. Your body is important—of course it is. But the most perfect body without a true mind and loving heart is nothing. Who you are inside determines how you relate to your body. Bodies can always be dressed up to feel attractive and sexy, but it's your mind and heart that determine the definition of attractive and sexy. When you understand and allow that belief to exude from you, you are one sassy woman!

WISE WOMAN WAYS

When I became a Reiki teacher, part of my training was developing the **hui yin** (Chinese for perineum) chakra, which is located between the anus and vagina. A fantastic side effect of learning to work with this area is greater pleasure and satisfaction when making love—for myself, but especially for my husband.

The old crone syndrome

Sometimes you may find yourself contemplating the "threat" of younger women, or comparing yourself to other women. We've got several schools near where I live, and going out in the early morning, at lunchtime, or around 3.30pm means engaging with a tide of nubile schoolgirls. Believe me, walking into an oncoming flow of girls wearing tight mini-skirts and sporting flawless skin, bouncing chests, and cascading hair means that a menopausal woman must make peace with herself as she is now and clearly embrace the virtues of getting older: seasoned attractiveness, worldly experience, and sexual mystery.

The loving art of masturbation

I believe that understanding our own sexuality through self-pleasuring is a stepping stone to being in sexual union with another. When we are in relationship, there are three energies; you, the other person, and the energy created by the union of the two. The same is true of the sexual act. There is your sexual relationship with yourself, your partner with themselves, and the energy created by the two. The more you can understand yourself, the more confident you will be in union with another. Allow yourself to have time on your own for self-discovery of your yoni area. Explore your own sensuality by exploring your entire body and it will open your mind to new possibilities. You could also do this with a partner, each of you taking turns to self-pleasure.

What Happens Next?

Expressing your sexuality is woven into Wise Woman ways. Creating ritual is also part of your menopausal healing. Let's find out how you might blend this sacred art into your journey.

CHAPTER 9

Creating Rituals

Rituals provide us with a sense of security and stability—from planting the spring bulbs to celebrating Yuletide. Ritual is different to habit. Habit, such as walking the dog, can be mindless but necessary, while ritual is an intentional, focused action. Ritual can create significance and celebration throughout the menopause years and offers opportunities to create harmony, patience, and appreciation in our lives.

Creating Sacred Space

Space is all around us. It can be full or empty. It can be literal (the kitchen) or abstract (our mind). Sacred can mean a special place to commune with yourself and the divine, whether it be God, Goddess, or something else. It is a space to be treated with reverence, set apart from the mundane. We can create a sacred space anywhere we choose—inside a building or outside in nature.

Casting your circle of sacred space

What we are doing when we cast a circle of sacred space is defining an area to be used for contemplation, meditation, or healing. This is the method I use when I am creating a sacred space. You can adapt it to suit your own needs:

1. Cleanse your area of work by, for example, smudging the area, using your besom (broom) to symbolically clear away negativity, or "singing bowls" to clear the space.
2. Ground and protect yourself.

3. Have everything inside your circle that you are likely to need.

4. Stand facing outwards at the eastern point. Place your hands together at the heart chakra, and bring your hands up to a point above your head as far as you can go. Say (silently or otherwise): "Guardian of the East and the element of Air, I call upon your presence and protection during this sacred healing." As you say the words, draw your hands apart in a wide circle until they meet palms and fingertips together at your second (sacral/spleen) chakra. Walk to the southern point.

5. Stand facing outwards at the southern point. Place your hands together at the heart chakra, and bring your hands up to a point above your head as far as you can go. Say (silently or otherwise): "Guardian of the South and the element of Fire, I call upon your presence and protection during this sacred healing." As you say the words, draw your hands apart in a wide circle until they meet palms and fingertips together at your second (sacral/spleen) chakra. Walk to the western point.

6. Stand facing outwards at the western point. Place your hands together at the heart chakra, and bring your hands up to a point above your head as far as you can go. Say (silently or otherwise): "Guardian of the West and the element of Water, I call upon your presence and protection during this sacred healing." As you say the words, draw your hands apart in a wide circle until they meet palms and fingertips together at your second (sacral/spleen) chakra. Walk to the northern point.

7. Stand facing outwards at the northern point. Place your hands together at the heart chakra, and bring your hands up to a point above your head as far as you can go. Say (silently or otherwise): "Guardian of the North and the element of Earth, Lord and Lady/God and Goddess, I call upon your presence and protection during this sacred healing." As you say the

words, draw your hands apart in a wide circle until they meet palms and fingertips together at your second (sacral/spleen) chakra. Walk to the eastern point.

8. Stand facing inwards at the eastern point, and point from where you are with the index finger of your dominant hand or with a crystal wand. Trace a clockwise circle of protection around you (and the other person if appropriate) or altar. Visualize the circle strong and protective around you, going deep down into the Earth and upwards to the sky. Ask the God and Goddess (or your choice) that all within the circle come under the full protection of the God and Goddess at all times.

9. When the circle is complete with your energy, you should declare what the circle is for. A statement that this circle is created in love and compassion for self-healing, for example.

WISE WOMAN WAYS

I find a certain amount of comfort in ritual. Maybe, it's the familiarity and safety that allow creative energy to build. However, it's also true that stepping into the energetic abyss armed with good grounding and protection can invite a level of inspiration unavailable when dealing with the purely familiar.

Having cast your circle, you must always close it after your work is complete. This is the method I use. You can adapt it to suit your needs:

1. Stand facing outwards at the eastern point. Place your hands together at the heart chakra, and bring your hands up to a point above your head as far as you can go. Say (silently or otherwise): "Guardian of the East and the element of Air,

I thank you for your presence and protection during this sacred healing. I bid you farewell." As you say the words, draw your hands apart in a wide circle until they meet palms and fingertips together at your second (sacral/spleen) chakra. Walk to the southern point.

2. Stand facing outwards at the southern point. Place your hands together at the heart chakra, and bring your hands up to a point above your head as far as you can go. Say (silently or otherwise): "Guardian of the South and the element of Fire, I thank you for your presence and protection during this sacred healing. I bid you farewell." As you say the words, draw your hands apart in a wide circle until they meet palms and fingertips together at your second (sacral/spleen) chakra. Walk to the western point.

3. Stand facing outwards at the western point. Place your hands together at the heart chakra, and bring your hands up to a point above your head as far as you can go. Say (silently or otherwise): "Guardian of the West and the element of Water, I thank you for your presence and protection during this sacred healing. I bid you farewell." As you say the words, draw your hands apart in a wide circle until they meet palms and fingertips together at your second (sacral/spleen) chakra. Walk to the northern point.

4. Stand facing outwards at the northern point. Place your hands together at the fourth (heart) chakra, and bring your hands up to a point above your head as far as you can go. Say (silently or otherwise): "Guardian of the North and the element of Earth, God and Goddess (or your choice), I thank you for your presence and protection during this sacred healing. I bid you farewell." As you say the words, draw your hands apart in a wide circle until they meet palms and finger-

tips together at your second (sacral/spleen) chakra. Walk to the eastern point.

5. Stand facing inwards at the eastern point, and point from where you are with your dominant hand, palm down and fingers outstretched, or use a crystal wand. Trace an anti-clockwise circle around you and the other person or altar. Visualize the circle melting around you.

Although I have done many rituals in a modest way, I was nervous about casting my first circle. In fact, only after a dream where I was casting a circle did I begin doing it for real. Even now, I am private in my rituals. A couple of years ago, I was doing a ritual alone in the garden, arms outstretched upwards—going great guns. I heard a noise behind me and saw my husband who had come home early from work, sitting quietly watching me. Although I know Mick has great respect for my beliefs, I still found it difficult when I knew he was watching.

Creating your personal altar as sacred space

An altar helps set your focus for menopausal rituals, ceremonies, and healing. This space should be large enough for you to conduct your work upon. It might be a permanent table or a table you put up and take down for use anywhere. I have "spaces" rather than altars. For example, there are spaces in my healing room for crystals. There are feathers in almost every room—small feathers in ceramic containers or large feathers amongst the plants. On the nightstand next to my side of the bed is an amethyst crystal with some night-time Rescue Remedy, plus a homeopathic remedy (all energy medicine). When the mood takes me, I put some flowers and greenery from the garden there as well, so the last thing I see at night is nature (or my lovely husband or maybe one of my four black cats peering down at me!).

You may choose to represent the four elements on your altar or sacred space with the following suggested articles:

- AIR: candles, feathers, smudge stick
- FIRE: candle, incense, a small cauldron, smudge stick, an oil burner, a vessel on which to burn herbs
- WATER: floating candle, flowers in water, a ritual chalice containing water
- EARTH: plant, a small branch, crystals/gems, a vessel on which to burn herbs

Before you begin any ritual, you should cleanse the area where the work is to be done and then cast the circle, as noted above. Once your work is complete, shut down the energy used for your workings, as discussed earlier, by thanking the guides, teachers, or God/Goddess that you called or who came into the circle to offer assistance. Then imagine the energy around the circle lowering around you and fading. Finally, clear the space with a blessing and ask the energies to close the spiritual gateways.

WISE WOMAN WAYS

Ritual for Aura Cleansing

Do the following exercise before going to bed at night or if you have been exposed to negative or scattered energy:

- Using the third and fourth fingers of both hands, press firmly on the point between the eyebrows. From there, with the same fingers, trace a line over the crown of the head and down to the back of the neck and then down the spine as far as you can reach.

- Still using the same fingers, reach under your arms and around to the centre of your back to pick up at the point you left off in step 1 and continue, pressing firmly down the centre of the back, the backs of the legs (simultaneously) to the calves. Finish with a flick of the fingers.
- With the third and fourth fingers of the right hand, start again at the point between the eyebrows and trace a line up and over the crown, down the back of the neck, back under your right side of your chin and along the left shoulder and the front of the left arm. Finish the movement with a sharp flick.
- Repeat the above, this time using the third and fourth fingers of the left hand and tracing the line over the head and down the front of the right arm.
- Using both hands, trace the line up from the point between the eyebrows over the head to the back of the neck. Here the hands separate, down each side of the neck under the jaw line, over the front of the throat, to join again at the breastbone. In one continuous flowing movement and maintaining firm pressure, follow the centre line down the front of the body with both hands and then (simultaneously), down both legs, finishing at the ankles, once again with a flick.

Rituals and Menopause

Although many women feel satisfaction in nourishing others, as our reproductive years come to a close it is appropriate to turn away from caretaking others to taking care of ourselves.

Wise Woman's time away

As the menopause years make themselves felt, we need to have time alone, where we free ourselves from responsibility to nourish and revision ourselves. Some ways in which the wise woman may do this:

- Prepare good food and eat mindfully.
- Engage in daily nature breaks.
- Restore rest periods during the day.
- Identify what you are willing to take on in order to reach your goals and what you are willing to let go of. Let go of relationships that do not enrich your life. Let go of possessions that do not enhance your life on a regular basis. Let go of things that take up space, require maintenance, and make decision-making more complicated. Let go of important tasks that someone else can do. Let go of petty annoyances. Make a list of 10 things in your life that bother you, then give yourself a month to fix it, clean it, toss it... Or let go of it—let go of the past.
- Indulge in regular child's play. Indulge in a craft project. Sit quietly and daydream.
- Begin your weekly planning by considering the activities you choose to care for your physical, spiritual, mental, and social well-being. Caring first for yourself helps you to be more available to serve in each of your chosen roles without resentment.
- Walk, exercise, or do some yoga. Enjoy a massage. Take a sauna. Get your hair done. Have a facial, pedicure, or manicure. Take a warm bath by candlelight before snuggling down in bed.

Ritual for Creating a Wise Woman Ceremony

Do you want to create a ceremony for perimenopause, menopause, or postmenopause? Why do you want to mark it? If you would like to enable healing, what healing and why? If you wish to strengthen and solidify a relationship, what kind of relationship and how do you want to strengthen or solidify it? Maybe you need to create a ceremony to remember what and why? It could be that you would like to state your beliefs and express your hope for the future. What beliefs? What are your hopes?

Preparing for the ceremony

Where would you like the ceremony? Who would you like to witness the ceremony? Do you want any special clothing?

Opening the ceremony

You might like to include candle lighting, music, essential oils or incense, a blessing, or a statement of intent.

Main body of the ceremony

You might like to include candle lighting, blessing of liquid/food, chanting, drumming, meditation, essential oils or incense, hand or foot washing, planting something, making a gift of charity, making a vow of service, reading text, storytelling, exchanging or giving gifts, creating amulets, singing, music, dancing, prayers and blessings, immersion in water, anointing, guided meditation or visualization, silence, the use of ritual objects.

Closing the ceremony

You could close with a blessing, music or sharing of food and drink

WISE WOMAN WAYS

Stand naked in front of a mirror by candlelight and create your anointing oil by mixing pure olive oil with frankincense or sandalwood. Ground and protect yourself and cast your sacred space. Take a drop of your mixture on your index finger and touch each chakra in turn while saying the following aloud:

- **CROWN**: Bless me, Dark Goddess, that my spirit may be clear and true.
- **THIRD EYE**: Bless my inner vision, that I may see with insight.
- **THROAT**: Bless my self-expression, that I may speak with wisdom.
- **HEART**: Bless my heart, that it be open and filled with compassion.
- **SOLAR PLEXUS**: Bless my sense of self-esteem, that I may be true to myself.
- **SACRAL**: Bless my womb, that I may always connect with my creative source.
- **ROOT**: Bless my yoni, the gateway of life and death.
- **BOTTOMS OF FEET**: Bless my feet, that I may symbolically walk my path with courage.
- **PALMS OF HANDS**: Bless my hands, that I may symbolically give and take with love.

What Happens Next?

Rituals are a creative way to honor the menopause years. We may choose not to use any tool in our ritual other than words and energy healing. However, we might choose to use nature's gift of the quartz crystals in our rituals. In the next chapter, let me tell you how you might do this.

CHAPTER 10

Using Quartz Crystals During Menopause

The composition of the earth is one-third quartz crystal and is one of the most abundant compounds found in the earth's surface and in most sedimentary, metamorphic, and igneous rocks. Quartz has also been found in lunar rocks. Did you know:

- The silica and water that crystals are composed of are also major components of the physical body?
- Quartz is fossilized water, and our bodies are 65-75 percent water?
- Crystals' piezoelectric effects (their energy fields) matches the earth's magnetic field and the magnetic field of the human aura?

There is a huge variety of quartz and quartz derivatives, including the following: agate, amethyst, ametrine, aqua aura quartz, aventurine, black quartz, bloodstone, blue siberian quartz, candle quartz, carnelian, cathedral quartz, chalcedony, chrysoprase, citrine, clear quartz, drusy quartz, elestial quartz, faden quartz, fairy quartz, golden healer quartz, green siberian quartz, heliotrope, jasper, lavender quartz, lepidocrosite herkimer, metamorphosis quartz, onyx, opal, phantom quartz, rock crystal, rose quartz, ruby aura quartz, rutilated quartz, sardonyx, smoky quartz, snow quartz, spirit quartz, starseed quartz, quartz, tiger's eye, and tourmaline.

You can find quartz in many everyday items, including sandpaper, soap, ceramics, radios, and televisions. It was the first crystal used in radio wave transceivers, is used in watches and timepieces, and was essential in the development of computers. When a crystal is put in a watch, the battery sends a constant charge through the crystal. The crystal absorbs the charge and then releases it at such a precise rate it is used to make the watch keep perfect time.

How Crystal Healing Works

The ancient Egyptians used lapis lazuli, turquoise, carnelian, emerald, and clear quartz in their jewellery and grave amulets. Stones were used for protection and health. A hieroglyphic papyrus from 2,000 B.C. documents a medical cure using crystal, and several from 1,500 B.C. have additional prescriptions.

Jade was seen as the concentrated essence of love and was recognized as a kidney healing stone both in China and South America. The original settlers of North, Central, and South America used crystals widely for spiritual, ceremonial, and healing purposes. Mayan Indians used quartz crystals for both the diagnosis and treatment of disease.

In Europe, from the 11th century through the Renaissance, a number of medical treatises appeared (Hildegard von Bingen, Arnoldus Saxo, and John Mandeville), extolling the virtues of precious and semiprecious stones in the treatment of ailments alongside herbal remedies.

The solar temple at Newgrange in the Boyne Valley of Ireland is older than the pyramids and was built so that the sun would stream through the 70-foot-long entrance tunnel on the Winter Solstice. Its roof was originally covered with white quartz,[25] to symbolize the White Goddess.

Quartz crystals focus, structure, amplify, transmit, transform, and store energy because they:

- have an energy grid of their own that evolves;
- absorb the energy of the earth, nature, environment, events,

and people around them and reveal their layers in response to different energies;

- have layers of growth and experience, as we do;
- and have their own karmic cycles.

American research scientist Marcel Vogel (1917–1991) worked for IBM for 27 years and developed the magnetic coating for IBM's disc drive and the first liquid crystal displays (LCD). He believed that the inner structure of crystals is in a perfect state of balance and radiates energy in a coherent manner that could be used to heal negative thought forms underlying disease. Macel also designed the vogel crystal,[26] which focuses the universal life force.

Crystals affect our electromagnetic energy fields, the subtle bodies that surround and permeate the physical body. A quartz crystal may be held in the hand and the healing energies sent through the palm chakra. As the energies pass through the crystal, they are both amplified and directed to the part of the subtle anatomy that requires energetic healing. Crystals complement other healing modalities. When placed on or around the body during a healing session and used in conjunction with other healing modalities, such as shamanic healing or Reiki, the crystals work both independently and cooperatively on healing.

Crystals needn't be held in order to experience their energies. They may be worn, placed in an environment (outside or inside), or even used in a distance healing capacity.

> **WISE WOMAN WAYS**
> I've always felt crystals, flowers, plants, herbs, and wood need to be placed together and try to do this aesthetically in the home as part of the décor.

Cleansing Crystals

Cleansing is the process of removing any previous energies and influences that a crystal may have either absorbed or come into contact with, either during its production, handling, or environment of origin. It is a good idea to cleanse the crystals you work with on a regular basis.

Water

Place the crystal in a clear glass bowl filled with water. CAUTION: Some crystals are water-soluble, which means they can dissolve in water. Most water-soluble crystals end in "ite." Fluorite, selinite, calcite, malachite, halite, sodolite, and rhodizite should all be kept away from water. Lapis lazuli, turquoise, ivory, and gypsum are also water-soluble. If you are not sure if your crystals are water-soluble, take a specimen and a steel knife. Scratch the surface. If it scratches, it is best to keep it out of water.

Salt

Most members of the quartz family are safe with salt, but some are not, including malachite, pyrite, angelite, some marbles and pearls, selenite, and opals. Dissolve one teaspoon of sea salt in one pint of water and place your crystal in the water overnight. Make sure you rinse all traces of salt away from the crystal and allow the crystal to dry naturally. Or you can bury your crystal in a bowl of natural sea salt for eight hours. Make sure you brush away all remains of salt.

Smudging

You can smudge crystals with sage, myrrh, sandalwood, frankincense, lavender, cedar, thyme, rosemary, or sweetgrass to cleanse them. Either fan the incense over the crystals with a feather or pass the crystal through the smoke of burning herbs, incense, or essential oil several times.

Other crystals

You can cleanse your crystal by placing it on a large crystal cluster for several hours. Quartz clusters are self-cleaning and charging. Citrine is also a cleansing crystal in its own right.

Sunlight

You can cleanse your crystals by placing them in direct sunlight, inside or out (sunlight is said to represent male energies). CAUTION: The sun will fade many crystals, including amethyst. Direct hot sun beaming through clear quartz may also be a fire hazard.

Moonlight

The moon can also cleanse crystals and is said to represent female energies. During the full moon, the moon's energy is enhanced and is a good time for cleaning crystals. Place the crystals outside or inside. CAUTION: If placing crystals outside, protect them from rain. I've cleansed crystals this way many times and find it a wonderful experience. We have a very long, terraced garden, which slopes away from the house. Sometimes I've placed the crystals out at dusk, so I don't break my neck getting down the garden at night. I have placed extra protection around the crystal layout, and not once have I found any crystal missing or out of place the next morning (no matter what the fairies and foxes may do at night!).

Intent

Hold your crystal in your hands and imagine a golden light from above coming down and filling the crystal and cleansing it of all negativity.

Sound

All crystals love sound, and you can use a tuning fork, singing bowl, or Tibetan cymbals to cleanse your crystals. Play your chosen sound over and around your crystal. This is a useful technique for large crystals. You might place one crystal inside a singing bowl.

Reiki

If you are attuned to Reiki you can use it to cleanse your crystals. This can be done by placing the crystals in your hands or holding your hands over the crystal and asking the Reiki to flow to cleanse the crystal. This is also a handy technique for any large or awkward crystals.

WISE WOMAN WAYS
Crystal Cave Meditation

Sit or lie comfortably. Close your eyes. Relax your body and slow your breathing. Imagine walking up a woodland path in the spring sunshine. As you walk, the path becomes progressively steeper. As you come to the crest of the hill, you see an opening to your left, leading to a cave in the side of the hill, partially hidden by flowering bushes. Walk into the cave. The air is cool and you see a sparkle where the walls are covered with black opals and red carnelian, giving off a scarlet glow. Walk through the cave of rich red crystals, absorbing their light. You move into another cave. Slowly, the opals and carnelian give way to tangerine quartz glowing a vibrant orange. Walk through the tangerine quartz, absorbing their light. You're moving deeper down into the earth and into another cave. Slowly, the tangerine quartz gives way to citrine and golden tiger's eye, shining with a sunshiny yellow. Walk through the citrine and golden tiger's eye, absorbing their light. The citrine and golden tiger's eye give way to a cave of rose quartz and rainforest jasper.

Walk through the crystals, absorbing their light. The crystals give way to a cave of turquoise crystals. Walk through the turquoise, absorbing its light. The turquoise gives way to walls of blue tiger's eye. Walk through the crystal cave, absorbing their light. Farther down and deeper you go. The crystals give way to an amethyst cave. Walk through the amethyst, absorbing its light. Finally, you walk into the innermost cavern, which is completely covered in pure rock crystal. Sit for a while in harmony with the healing crystals and the quiet stillness of the earth before returning to the outer world.

Charging Crystals

You will need to recharge your crystals immediately after cleaning them. While your crystal already contains its own unique vibrational energies, those energies can sometimes become low or depleted. When you recharge crystals, you're basically giving them the chance to refresh their ability to focus and expand their energy.

Crystal clusters

Crystal cluster chunks, or caves, are known to be self-charging and will charge other crystals lain upon them.

Sound

Put a crystal near a single-note chime and strike the chime gently several times. This has a harmonizing effect on the crystal. If you like to chant, do so in the presence of your crystals. Put your crystal near a bell and gently produce a sound in it. Instead of using a bell you can use a resonant (tune) fork.

Reiki charging

If you are a Reiki practitioner, you can charge your crystals with Reiki energy.

Sunlight

The ultraviolet light from the sun containing the full spectrum of light restores a crystal's energy. CAUTION: The sun will fade many crystals, such as amethyst. Direct hot sun beaming through clear quartz may also be a fire hazard.

Moonlight

Crystals can be recharged using the softened solar radiation reflected via the moon. CAUTION: If placing outside, protect your crystals from rain.

> **WISE WOMAN WAYS**
>
> I have to confess to occasionally needing to cleanse and charge my crystals when I do not have a lot of time to spare. As long as your intent is honourable and clear, it's wonderful how quickly the crystals will oblige! The crystals I have the privilege of working with may be used for teaching or healing. I offer a prayer for protection and of intent, asking that the crystals be cleansed of all negative energy and charged with the blessings of the Goddess for the highest good of all. I then smudge the room and the crystals.

Chakra Balancing with Crystals

One of the simplest ways to use crystals during the menopause years is to balance the chakra system using crystals. To realign chakra energies, place one or two crystal of the appropriate colour on each chakra area for a few minutes.

First (root or base) chakra

How it can help: This will balance physical energy, motivation, and practicality and promote a sense of reality. It's a good idea to place a grounding stone like smoky quartz or black tourmaline between the feet to act as an anchor.

Related quartz crystals: Red tourmaline, black opal, onyx, red aventurine, red carnelian, red chalcedony, red phantom quartz, red-brown agate, ruby aura quartz, rutilated quartz, black smoky quartz, grey banded and botswanna agate, heliotrope, rainbow jasper, red and brecciated jasper, and red tiger's eye.

Second (sacral or spleen) chakra

How it can help: This will balance creativity and release blocks in your life that prevent pleasure.

Related quartz crystals: Carnelian, bushmen red cascade quartz, carnelian agate, drusy quartz, fire agate, fire opal, harlequin quartz, lepidocrosite included in quartz or amethyst, orange phantom quartz, Oregan opal, reversed orange phantom quartz, tangerine quartz, red jasper, and chryoprase.

Third (solar plexus) chakra

How it can help: To reduce anxiety, clear thoughts, and improve confidence.

Related quartz crystals: Citrine, spirit quartz, lemon chryoprase, opal aura quartz, smokey citrine, snakeskin agate, sunshine aura quartz, yellow jasper, yellow phantom quartz, yellow tourmaline, sulphur in quartz, golden healer quartz, rutilated quartz, and golden tiger's eye.

Fourth (heart) chakra

How it can help: To promote a sense of calm, create a sense of direction in life, and balance your relationship with others and the world.

A pink stone can be added for emotional clearing.

Related quartz crystals: Aventurine, apple aura quartz, chryoprase, dentric agate, epidote in quartz, green agate, green aventurine, green jasper, helitrope, leopardskin jasper (jaguar stone), moss agate, ocean orbicular jasper (the Atlantis stone), olive jasper, peach aventurine, pink agate, pink carnelian, pink chalcedony, pink crackle quartz, pink phantom quartz, pink tourmaline, prasiolite (green quartz), rainforest jasper, rose aura quartz, Siberian green quartz, smokey rose quartz, strawberry quartz, green tourmaline, and rose quartz.

Fifth (throat) chakra

How it can help: To bring peace, ease communication difficulties, and promote self-expression.

Related quartz crystals: Aqua aura, Andean blue opal, aura quartz, blue aventurine, blue chalcedony, blue jasper, blue lace agate, blue phantom quartz, blue tiger's eye, blue-green agate, flame aura quartz, girasol (blue opal), indicolite (blue tourmaline), moss agate, rainbow aura quartz, Siberian blue quartz, tourmaline, water opal (hyalite), watermelon tourmaline, avalonite (drusy blue chalcedony), and blue agate.

Sixth (brow) chakra

How it can help: To promote intuitive skills and memory and increase understanding and self-knowledge.

Related quartz crystals: Amethyst, blue jasper, blue tiger's eye, chrysophal (blue-green opal) smoky quartz, and moss agate.

Seventh (crown) chakra

How it can help: This will integrate and balance all aspects of the self—physical, mental, emotional, and spiritual—and will promote positive thought patterns, inspiration, and imagination.

Related quartz crystals: Amethyst, amethyst elestial, amethyst herkimer, amethyst phantom quartz, amethyst spirit quartz, Botswana agate, brandenberg amethyst, lavender quartz, lavender amethyst, lithium quartz, purple jasper, purple tourmaline, purple violet tourmaline, rock crystal, royal plume jasper, smokey amethyst, titanium quartz, vera cruz amethyst, violet amethyst, ametrine, and clear quartz.

WISE WOMAN WAYS
Chakra Balancing Meditation
Choose one or more stones for each chakra. Lie down and place each stone on the appropriate location. Hold a clear quartz point and rotate it over each stone, beginning at the first chakra. Inhale deeply. As you inhale, imagine your breath coming up through the earth and through the soles of your feet, filling your body as it rises to the top of your head and comes out like a fountain. As you exhale, imagine it travelling back down over your body and sinking into the earth.

Crystals for Different Menopausal States

Menopausal State	Quartz Crystal
Aging issues	Rose quartz, rutilated quartz, boulder opal
Apprehension, anxiety, stress, worry	Amethyst, aventurine, clear quartz, rose quartz, smoky quartz, black tourmaline, blue lace agate, watermelon, tourmaline, carnelian, green aventurine, Herkimer diamond, siberian quartz, jasper, fire agate,

	smoky quartz, jasper (chakras: brow, heart, solar plexus)
Constipation	Smoky quartz, black tourmaline
Depression	Amethyst, celestial quartz, smoky quartz, rose quartz, carnelian, amethyst, smoky quartz, black tourmaline, rutilated quartz, lithium quartz, ametrine, Botswana agate, carnelian, moss agate, tiger's eye, purple tourmaline, Siberian quartz (chakra: solar plexus)
Excessive bleeding	Jasper, carnelian (chakras: solar plexus, root/base)
Excess weight	Dream quartz
Fatigue	Clear quartz, yellow jasper, black tourmaline, peru opal, amethyst, rose quartz, carenelian, fire agate, ametrine, blue opal, dendritic agate (chakra: root/base)
Fuzzy thinking, lack of concentration	Clear quartz, black tourmaline, amethyst, smoky quartz, opal, moss agate, green tourmaline, red jasper (chakras: brow, crown)
Grounding	Jasper, smoky quartz
Hot flushes	Ametrine, smoky quartz, moonstone, chrysocolla, citrine, blue tourmaline, fire agate, rose quartz
Indecisive, self-doubting	Carnelian, smoky quartz, tiger's eye
Insomnia	Amethyst, smoky quartz, candle quartz, moonstone, chrysoprase,

	rose quartz (chakra: brow)
Intolerant, critical, irritable	Rose quartz
Low self-esteem	Rose quartz, moss agate, chryso-beryl, citrine, opal, tourmaline (chakras: root, spleen/sacral, heart)
Lack of sexual interest	Carnelian, rose quartz (chakra: brow, root/base, spleen/sacral, heart)
Low vitality	Black tourmaline, fire opal, rutilated quartz, carnelian
Panic	Green tourmaline
Passivity	Chrysoprase, tiger's eye
Sadness, loss (of youth)	Red jasper
Anger	Black tourmaline, chrysocolla, moss and green tree agate, rose quartz, chyrsoprase (chakra: root/base)

WISE WOMAN WAYS

Massaging with crystals combines the relaxing benefits of massage with the healing energy of crystals. If feeling stressed or headachy, choose smooth clear quartz crystals such as spheres (I use the smooth end of a wand, one for either side of the head), tumble stones, or palm stones. Circle the crystal gently around the temples and over the forehead.

Ways to Use Crystals

In grids

A crystal grid involves using six single-pointed crystals (I would suggest using clear quartz or amethyst). If you are laying down, place one by your left foot with the point going up, one by your elbow, point up, and one by the left of your head point up. Then place one by the right of your head point going down, one by your elbow, point down, and one by your right foot, point down.

Placement of the Crystals

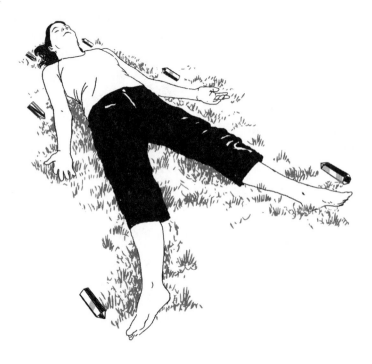

If you are sitting in a chair, place a crystal by your left foot going up, one just behind the chair on your left going up, one just behind the chair on your right going down, and one by your right foot, going down. You may choose to hold a crystal in your hand.

Gem essences

Gem essences can be dropped under the tongue, rubbed into pulse or chakra points, sprayed into the aura, put in bath water, or sprayed around a room. The basic principle behind the use of gem essences is the same as that of flower essences, in that when crystals are activated by natural sunlight or moonlight, they transfer their vibrational signature into water, creating a remedy that is safe and can be used in conjunction with all healing modalities. Once you have your gem essence, you can enhance it with flower essences. Put two drops of the chosen flower essences into the gem mixture. This is a particularly nice way to blend the energies of Bach Flower Remedies or Australian Bush Flower Essences with crystals. CAUTION: Some gems are toxic when taken directly into the body.

Other ways to use crystals

You could wear a crystal, place it under your pillow, or hold it while meditating. Experiment with placing crystals at strategic points in a room.

> **WISE WOMAN WAYS**
> Make up a crystal power pouch containing the crystals of your choice, plus some sage for cleansing negativity, and carry it with you.

What Happens Next?

Crystals are a gift to you from Mother Earth and can be used as part of your energy healing during the menopause years. Another Wise Woman healing art that uses energy healing is hand reflexology, which you can easily learn and do anywhere to help comfort and sooth any distress of menopause. Interested to know more? Then turn the page and read on.

CHAPTER 11

Hand Reflexology for Menopause

Whilst the art of reflexology dates back to Ancient Egypt, India, and China, it wasn't until 1913 that Dr. William Fitzgerald[27] introduced this therapy to the West as Zone Therapy. Dr Fitzgerald researched how reflex areas on the feet and hands were linked to areas and organs of the body within the same zone. During the 1930s, Eunice Ingham[28] further developed this zone theory into what is now known as reflexology, observing that congestion in any part of the foot was mirrored in the corresponding part of the body.

What Is Hand Reflexology?

The feet are rich in nerve endings, which is why they are traditionally used by reflexologists to stimulate the flow of energy throughout the body, but the hands (and other key areas of the body) can also be used successfully, as discussed below. Hand reflexology can be self-administered anywhere and can bring ease and comfort during the menopausal years.

Hand reflexology contraindications

The main hand reflexology contraindications are as follows:

- Don't do it on broken skin or if there are infected sores or lesions on the hands.
- Don't do hand reflexology if you have a hand injury.
- If you have any medical problem, consult a doctor first.

If you can't use your fingers or knuckles, use the blunt end of a pencil or the blunt end of a crystal wand.

Hand reflexology techniques

You may use all these techniques in one session, or just one technique:

1. RUBBING: Briskly rubbing your palms together will generate energy (chi) in them. Rubbing is also part of the hand reflexology routine.
2. SQUEEZING: Using your thumb pad and index finger to firmly squeeze each finger and thumb on the other hand, from base to tip.
3. PULLING: Using your thumb pad and index finger to firmly grasp the base of each finger and thumb on the other hand and pull down towards the tip.
4. PRESSING: Using the tip of your thumb to press and stimulate points on the opposite hand (you will need short nails!). Press until you feel pressure. Hold the pressure and work the point with rotary, or circular, pressure.
5. ROTARY, OR CIRCULAR, PRESSURE: Press into the point and move in very small firm circles using a knuckle of the other hand or the blunt end of a pencil or crystal wand. I would recommend a rose quartz wand or maybe amethyst with a little lavender oil on the blunt end (not too much or the wand will slip).
6. THUMB ROLL: Rolling the pad of your thumb over the points,

Massage the relevant points on both hands a couple of times a day. Hand pressure points adapt to stimulation, so after seven days stop for three days. If the symptoms persist, continue for another week (or more) or choose new points to press and work.

> **WISE WOMAN WAYS**
>
> You could put a flower essences mixture in the centre of your palms before giving yourself hand reflexology. Or mix a little lavender, rose, or geranium oil with some hand cream or oil and rub into your hands before giving yourself hand reflexology. Not too much, otherwise your fingers will skid everywhere!

Self-treatment

1. Begin your hand reflexology treatment by sitting quietly and closing your eyes. Take a few deep breaths as you still your body and focus your mind.

2. Begin your hand reflexology treatment by pinching the tips of each finger and thumb of your left hand (nail to back). Reverse and repeat this process on your right hand. The pressure applied to your fingers should be firm but not painful. A few seconds for each finger tip will do.

3. After pinching the tops your finger and thumb tips go back to each tip and pinch them again, this time squeezing from side to side.

4. Vigorously rub from base to tip of each finger and thumb of your left hand, front and back plus sides. Reverse and repeat this process on your right hand.

5. Tug each finger and thumb firmly.

6. Using your right thumb and forefinger, firmly grasp the webbed area between your thumb and forefinger of your left hand. Keeping a firm hold, tug at the skin gently until the fleshy web snaps away from your grasp. Repeat this process for the areas between all your fingers. Reverse and repeat this process on your right hand.

7. Turn your left hand palm down. Use your right thumb to massage the back of your hand. Massage the knuckles and in between

knuckle area first. Continue thumb massaging each area on the back of the hand. Reverse and repeat this process on your right hand.

8. Cradle your left wrist (palm up) inside your right hand. Use your thumb to massage your inner wrist. This is an especially soothing massage for anyone who routinely uses their wrists in repetitive movements, such as computer work. Reverse and repeat this process on your right hand.

9. Massage the palm of your left hand with your right thumb, knuckle, or the blunt end of a crystal wand. Massage the fleshier mound areas more deeply. Reverse and repeat this process on your right hand.

10. At the end of the session press your right thumb or the blunt end of a crystal wand deeply in the center of your left palm. Reverse and repeat this process on your right hand. Take a few deep breaths and center yourself.

> **WISE WOMAN WAYS**
> If you are a Reiki II or III practitioner, activate your hand chakras before giving yourself hand reflexology.

Specific Menopausal Points

ENDORPHIN STIMULATION: Find the pituitary gland on center of the thumbprint swirl on the left hand and apply rotary pressure on this point. Reverse and repeat this process on your right hand. Note: Avoid if pregnant.

EYESTRAIN: The eye reflex points are at the base of the index, middle, and ring fingers on the "big knuckles." Apply rotary pressure directly on these knuckles as well as just above and below the knuckles on both sides of both hands.

HOT FLUSHES: Find the hypothalamus gland just above the centre of the thumbprint swirl on the left hand and apply rotary pressure using the thumb of the right hand. Reverse and repeat this process on your right hand.

BACK PAIN: Work the spine points, which run along the outer edge of the thumb down towards the wrist. Apply rotary pressure along this area with the other hand. The point where the centre of your hand joins your wrist can be stimulated to give relief from lower back pain.

HORMONE BALANCE: Work the thyroid gland reflex on the left hand (under nail on thumb) using rotary pressure. Reverse and repeat this process on your right hand.

Work the ovary reflex on the left wrist (where the wrist and hand meet below little finger) by applying rotary pressure on the area using the thumb of the right hand. Reverse and repeat this process on your right hand. Use this point to improve sexual energy.

Work the uterus reflex on the left wrist (below thumb extending round wrist like a bracelet) by rubbing with your right thumb, using gentle but firm pressure on the area indicated (this reflex extends around the wrist like a bracelet). Reverse and repeat this process on your right hand. This could help ease menstruation difficulties, balance hormones, and improve libido.

BREAST TENDERNESS: Work the breast reflex on the left hand (top of hands under fingers) by rubbing using gentle but firm pressure using the thumb of the right hand. Reverse and repeat this process on your right hand.

SHOULDER PAIN: Part of the shoulder reflex is on both palms of the hand under the little finger, which can be worked with a rotary pressure. Working the reflex points on the backs of the hands in the grooves between the long bones will ease tension over and between the shoulder blades. To work them, use your fingertips. If your left shoulder is the problem, work the reflex points on your left hand.

Put your right thumb flat on your left palm. On the back of your left hand, place the tips of your right index, middle, and ring fingers in the grooves. Gently apply and maintain even pressure, slowly and repeatedly moving your fingertips in the direction of the wrist. Reverse and repeat on the right hand.

SINUS: Squeeze and pull around the sinus reflex points on the top third of each finger and thumb (completely around the finger and thumb) on both hands.

NECK DISCOMFORT: Work the reflex points on the top half of the left thumb. Thumb roll the area between the knuckle and nail of each thumb. Use the thumb or index knuckle of right hand moving slowly and firmly down the outside of the thumb nail to the knuckle, pressing all the way. Reverse and repeat on right hand.

BLADDER: With your left palm up, the bladder point is just above where the base of the thumb joins the wrist. Apply pressure to this point with your thumb or knuckle. Reverse and repeat on the right hand.

FATIGUE: Work the adrenal reflex on the left hand with your right. Find the webbing between thumb and index finger and go into the palm about an inch. Apply a rotary pressure on the area indicated using the thumb or knuckle of the right hand. Reverse and repeat this process on your right hand. Do not work this reflex if you have high blood pressure.

HEADACHES: Apply rotary pressure all around the nail area of the left thumb with your other hand. Reverse and repeat on the right hand

ANXIETY: Find the skin crease that runs right across your wrist at the base of your hand. The point is almost at the end of the crease, just inside the edge of the wrist bone (little finger side). Use your thumb pad to press the point until you feel a strong pressure. Hold the pressure while you knead the point using rotary movements for about 1 minute. Repeat on the other wrist. Press both points 2-3 times a day or and whenever you feel anxious.

The ears (like the feet and hands) contain reflexology points corresponding to major body parts and areas. Sit with your back straight. Use your thumbs and your index fingers to rub and gently pull your ears from the top to bottom. You can also use the tips of your index fingers to rub the inside surface of both ears. Start at the ear opening and work your way to the outside edge, rubbing all the curves and folds of each ear, including behind your ears. Do this for 1-2 minutes per ear.

Helpful Reflexology Points for Menopause

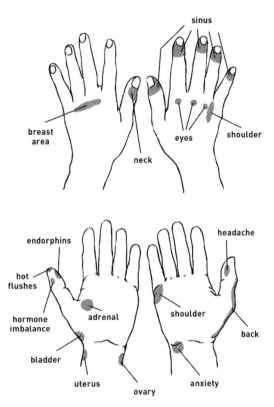

WISE WOMAN WAYS

Sometimes my lower back gets a little temperamental, so I use hand reflexology to ease the discomfort. I tend to use my knuckles (especially the corner of a knuckle), and I use very small movements as I move down the spinal area on the thumbs.

What Happens Next?

We have travelled through this book together and I hope you have reached this point with some inspiration for your own menopausal journey. Until we meet again.

Further Reading

Aubyn, Lorna St. *Everyday Rituals and Ceremonies*. London: Piatkus, 1998.

Baring, Anne and Jules Cashford. *The Myth of the Goddess: Evolution of an Image*. London: Arkana Penguin, 1993.

Capacchione, Lucia. *The Creative Journal*. Pompton Plains, NJ: New Page Books, 2002.

Conway D.J. *Maiden, Mother, Crone*. Woodbury, MN: Llewellyn Publications, 1994.

Crawford, Amanda McQuade. *The Herbal Menopause Book*. Freedom, CA: The Crossing Press, 1996.

Davis, Martha and Elizabeth Robbins Eshelman. *The Relaxation & Stress Reduction Workbook*. Oakland, CA: New Harbinger Publications, 2000.

Ewing, Jim Pathfinder. *Finding Sanctuary in Nature*. Forres, Scotland: Findhorn Press, 2007.

Gienger, Michael. *Crystal Massage for Health and Healing*. Forres, Scotland: Findhorn Press, 2006.

Gienger, Michael. *Healing Crystals*. Forres, Scotland: Findhorn Press, 2005.

Gienger, Michael and Joachim Goebel. *Gem Water*. Forres, Scotland: Findhorn Press, 2008.

Gray, Linda. *Grow Your Own Pharmacy*. Forres, Scotland: Findhorn Press, 2007.

Guhr, Andreas and Jorg Nagler. *Crystal Power: Mythology and History*. Forres, Scotland: Findhorn Press, 2006.

Harvey, Clare. *The New Encyclopedia of Flower Remedies*. London: Watkins Publishing, 2007.

Judith, Anodea and Slen Vega. *The Sevenfold Journey*. Freedom, CA: Crossing Press, 1993.

Keet, Michael and Louise. *Hand Reflexology: Stimulate Your Body's Healing System*. London: Hamlyn, 2004.

Kenton, Leslie. *Passage to Power*. London: Vermilion, 1999.

Kliegel, Ewald. *Crystal Wands*. Forres, Scotland: Findhorn Press, 2009.

Kynes Sandra. *Your Altar*. Woodbury, MN: Llewellyn Publications, 2007.

Linn, Denise. *Sacred Space*. London: Rider, 2005.

McCain, Marian Van Eyk. *Elderwoman*. Forres, Scotland: Findhorn Press, 2002.

Northrup, Dr Christiane. *The Wisdom of Menopause: Creating Physical and Emotional Health and Healing During the Change*. Revised Edition. London: Random House, 2009.

Reif, Jennifer and Marline Haleff. *The Magical Crone*. New York, NY: Citadel Press (Kensington Publishing), 2003.

Roads, Michael J. *Conscious Gardening*. Forres, Scotland: Findhorn Press, 2011.

Sarita, Mahasatvaa Ma Ananda. *Divine Sexuality*. Forres, Scotland: Findhorn Press, 2011.

Scheffer, Mechthild. *The Encyclopedia of Bach Flower Therapy*. Rochester, VT: Healing Arts Press (Bear and Co.), 2001.

Seaward, Brian Luke. *Stand Like Mountain, Flow Like Water*. Deerfield Beach, FL: HCI Books, 1997.

Silveira, Isabel. *Quartz Crystals*. Forres, Scotland: Findhorn Press, 2008.

Stewart, Maryon. *The Phyto Factor*. New York, NY: Random House, 2000.

Vennell, David. *Healing Hands: Simple and Practical Reflexology Techniques for Developing Good Health and Inner Peace*. Hants., UK: O Books (John Hunt Publishing), 2005.

Weed, Susun. *New Menopausal Years the Wise Woman Way*. Woodstock, NY: Ash Tree Publishing, 2002.

White, Ian. *Australian Bush Flower Essences*. Forres, Scotland: Findhorn Press, 1993.

Zinn, Jon Kabbat. *Wherever You Go There You Are: Mindfulness Meditation in Everyday Life*. London: Piatkus, 2004.

Endnotes

CHAPTER 1

1   John Carvel. "Post-menopause women 'happier'." *The Guardian.*
    2002. www.guardian.co.uk/uk/2002/may/08/research.health.
    Accessed on 12.6.11

2   "Facts and statistics about the baby boomer generation."
    Baby-Boomer magazine. www.babyboomer-magazine.com.
    Accessed on 13.6.11.

3   "Tamoxifen: Questions and Answers." National Cancer Institute
    at the National Institutes of Health. www.cancer.gov/cancertop-
    ics/factsheet/Therapy/tamoxifen. Accessed on 12.6.11.

4   "Early menopause: feeling good and finding your way." Marcelle
    Pick. 2011. Women-to-Women. www.womentowomen.com/
    menopause/earlymenopause.aspx. Accessed on 13.6.11.

5   "Psychological symptoms of menopause." Dr. Anita Houghton.
    www.menopausematters.co.uk/psychological.php. Accessed on
    13.6.11.

6   John Carvel. "Post-menopause women 'happier'." *The Guardian.*
    2002. www.guardian.co.uk/uk/2002/may/08/research.health.
    Accessed on 12.6.11

CHAPTER 2

7   "Hunter-gatherer." *New World Encylopedia.* 2008. www.newworl-
    dencyclopedia.org/entry/Hunter-gatherer#Structure_of_Hunter-
    gatherer_Societies. Accessed on 13.6.11.

8   "Venus of Willendorf." Christopher L. C. E. Witcombe, 2003.
    http://arthistoryresources.net/willendorf/willendorfdiscovery.
    html. Accessed on 13.6.11.

9   Walker, Barbara. *The Women's Encyclopedia of Myths and Secrets.*
    HarperSanFrancisco, 1987.

10   Harvey, Graham. *Listening People, Speaking Earth: Contempo-rary Paganism* (Second Edition). London: Hurst and Company, 2007, pp1-2.

11   Farrar, Janet and Farrar, Stewart. *The Witches' Goddess: The Feminine Principle of Divinity*. London: Robert Hale, 1987, pp 29-37.

12   "Names of the Goddess." Judith Q Addendum. *Mother Goddess*. www.mothergoddess.com. Accessed on 13.6.11.

CHAPTER 3

13   John R. Lee, MD. www.johnleemd.com. Accessed on 13.6.11.

14   "How to Obtain Natural Progesterone." The Natural Progesterone Information Service. www.npis.info/howtoobtain.htm. Accessed on 13.6.11.

15   Northrup, Dr. Christiane. *The Wisdom of Menopause*. Piatkus, 2009, pp 241-243

CHAPTER 4

16   The National Institute of Medical Herbalists. www.nimh.org.uk. Accessed on 13.6.11.

CHAPTER 5

17   The Bach Centre. www.bachcentre.com. Accessed on 13.6.11.

18   Australian Bush Flower Essences (ABFE). www.ausflowers.com.au. Accessed on 13.6.11.

CHAPTER 6

19   Siegelman, E. *Personal Risk: Mastering Change in Love and Work*. New York: Harper and Row, 1983.

20   Hales, D. *An Invitation to Health*. Belmont, CA: Wadsworth/Thomson Learning, 2003.

21   Kiecolt-Glaser, J.K., McGuire, L., Robles, T.F. and Glaser, R. (2002) "Psychoneuroimmunology: Psychological influences on

immune function and health." *Journal of Consulting and Clinical Psychology* 70, 3, 537–547. http://pni.osumc.edu/KG%20Publications%20%28pdf%29/150.pdf. Accessed on 1.6.11.

22   Spiegel, D. Stanford School of Medicine Centre on Stress and Health. http://stresshealthcenter.stanford.edu. Accessed on 6.12.10.

CHAPTER 8

23   Sarita, Mahasatvaa Ma Ananda. *Divine Sexuality*. Findhorn Press, 2011, pp89.

24   ———. *Divine Sexuality*. Findhorn Press, 2011, pp99

CHAPTER 10

25   www.newgrange.com. This site includes information on how white quartz might have been used in the mound or "cairn." Accessed on 23.6.11

26   Vogel Crystals. www.vogelcrystals.net/index.htm. Accessed on 23.06.11.

CHAPTER 11

27   "History: Dr William H Fitzgerald MD." Modern Institute of Reflexology. www.reflexologyinstitute.com/reflex_fitzgerald.php. Accessed on 13.6.11.

CHAPTER 11

28   "History of Reflexology." International Institute of Reflexology. www.reflexology-usa.net/history.htm. Accessed on 13.6.11.

FINDHORN PRESS

Life-Changing Books

For a complete catalogue,
please contact:

Findhorn Press Ltd
117-121 High Street,
Forres IV36 1AB,
Scotland, UK

t +44 (0)1309 690582
f +44 (0)131 777 2711
e info@findhornpress.com

or consult our catalogue online
(with secure order facility) on
www.findhornpress.com

For information on the Findhorn Foundation:
www.findhorn.org